FOURT

COLD WATER CURE,

ITS

PRINCIPLES, THEORY, AND PRACTICE;

WITH AMPLE

Directions for its Self-application;

AND

A FULL ACCOUNT OF THE WONDERFUL CURES PERFORMED WITH IT
ON 7,000 PATIENTS, OF ALL NATIONS.

BY THE DISCOVERER,

VINCENT PRIESSNITZ,

OF GRÄEFENBERG, IN SILESIA.

"In the midst of a society, where wine and spirits are considered as of little more value than water, I have lived two years without either; AND WITH NO OTHER DRINK BUT WATER, except when I have found it convenient to obtain milk; not an hour's illness; not a headach for an hour; not the smallest ailment; not a restless night; not a drowsy morning have I known during these two famous years of my life. The sun never rises before me, I have always to wait for him to come and give me light to write by, while my mind is in full vigour, and while nothing has come to cloud its clearness."—*Cobbett*.

"On ascending to Gräefenberg by the carriage road, the traveller will see a fountain erected by Wallachian and Moldavian patients, with this inscription:—

'V. P.
'TO THE GENIUS OF COLD WATER.'

"And on descending by the foot-path to Friewaldau, he will find another monument of a lion, on a pedestal, in bronze, erected by the Hungarians, with the following inscriptions in their language:—

FRONT.

'As a punishment to man for his presumption in despising the beverage which he had in common with wild animals, he became diseased, infirm, and debilitated.
'Priessnitz causes the primitive virtues of water to be again known, and by it infuses fresh vigour into the human race.'

SIDE.

'Priessnitz, the benefactor of mankind, merits the grateful and honourable remembrance of the Hungarian nation. The erectors of this monument invite their countrymen of future ages to the vivifying springs at Gräefenberg.
'MDCCCXXXIX et XL.'"
—Vide pages 41 & 42.

LONDON:
WILLIAM STRANGE, 21, PATERNOSTER ROW;
AND E. SMITH, 6, WELLINGTON STREET, STRAND.

1843.

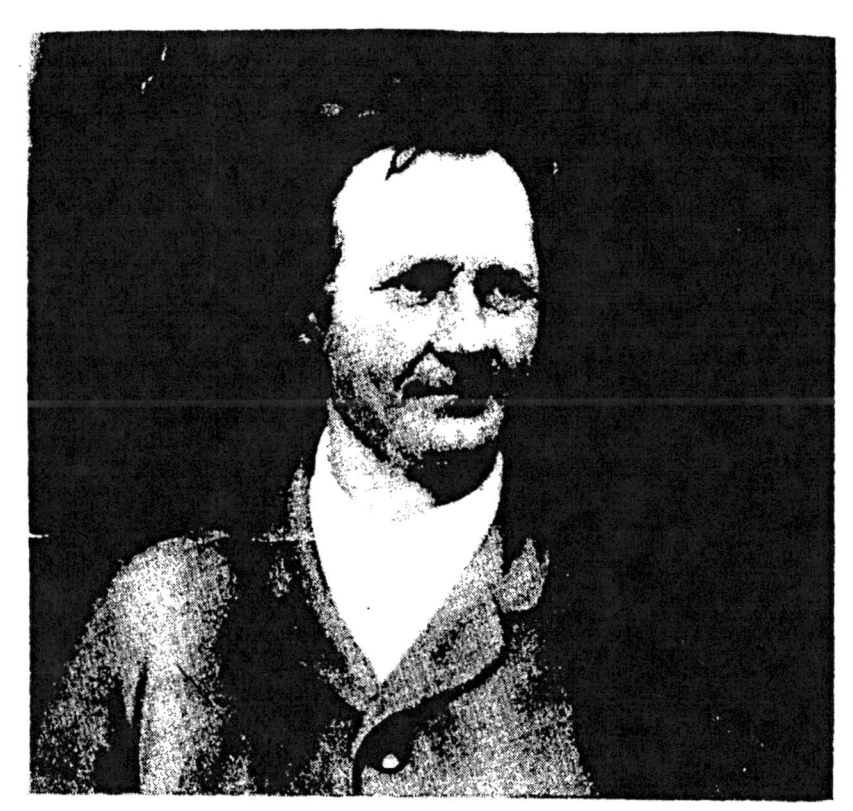

VINCENT PRIESSNITZ --
OCTOBER 4, 1799, NOVEMBER 28, 1851
FOUNDER AND INVENTOR OF THE
"WATER CURE"

Jesse Mercer Gehman, N.D.,D.C.,M.N.

Vincent Priessnitz was not the first man to use cold water to overcome disease. No doubt other men before him had made observations as did he and used it for the alleviation of pain and the dissolution of illness in the body. However, Vincent Priessnitz was the first man to formulate a complete system of cold water treatments for that purpose. His is the only name, of all the pioneers in the Nature Cure and Hygienic movement, preserved in medical dictionaries.

That Vincent Priessnitz made the discovery of the power of cold water in healing the ills of the body, and reached his conclusions independently of all other healers who preceded him there is not the slightest doubt.

Born of hard working country people at Grafenberg, Germany in upper Silesia, he led the life of the usual country boy. Scarcely less observing than he was industrious, he observed from his vantage point as his flock grazed, a wounded doe, injured by hunters, wade into the calm backflow waters of the turbulent mountain brook. He wondered as the doe limped away and disappeared into the forest. That night he decided there must be a reason for a wounded animal to seek water to lave its wounds. Perhaps instinct was stronger than reason. He would return the next day. He did.

Sure enough the doe returned to the eddying water at about the same time. It stood silently, without a move, and then after awhile limped to the bank and disappeared in the deep foliage of the forest once more. For two weeks the lad Vincent Priessnitz returned daily to his vantage point and watched. For two weeks the wounded doe returned and bathed its injured leg in the brook. Each day the deer walked better and finally scampered out of the water on the last day to return no more.

Before his very eyes he had seen a badly injured deer healed with cool sparkling brook water. Vincent Priessnitz never forgot that experience.

Some years later Priessnitz was injured severely hauling cord wood. Night stole upon him, as did a heavy snow storm. His team bolted through a gulch. The load slipped and his ribs were crushed.

But while he lay there he had time to reflect on what to do. A doctor was out of the question on a night like that. No help was forthcoming. Somehow he managed to get home.

No, he could not soak his injured ribs in water as the deer had done with its leg. He conceived the idea of wrapping the injured ribs with pieces of his torn shirt soaked in cold water. This relieved him. He continued to apply cold wet wrappings and in due course his ribs were free from pain and healed.

The news of his accomplishment spread. When a neighbor became injured he called for the young man who healed with water. Requests for aid became more frequent and further from home, and his experience grew apace.

He gave the matter of his discovery, which had meant so much to himself and others much thought. He tried various applications with varying degrees of success. Empirically by trial and error he evolved a method or system of cold water treatment that brought help to thousands.

He opened a modest place where people could stay. In a matter of months it became the haven of the sick. His fame spread to every corner of the globe. He treated Prince and pauper alike. The medical big wigs of the day protested and closed his doors. To his patients, called to the center of the square, he said: "be undismayed. If they will not let me use water we shall find a cure in air."

He was persecuted and prosecuted. By trickery and scheming the medical fraternity sought to discredit him. The people who had been healed were evidence against any wrong doing he was accused of. The final gesture was the claim that the water was drugged. The State found he used only pure mountain water.

To end all persecution the State decreed that no one should ever molest him, that he be permitted to heal the sick as he had been doing.

Grafenberg became a shrine for the ill. People traveled to it from all over the world. Some of the best records we have came from the pen of Americans who crossed the ocean to take the "cure."

In 1842, twelve hundred patients from all over the world visited and were cared for at his institution at Grafenberg. During the years 1849, 1850 and 1851, the number of patients rose to as high as fourteen hundred, and came from as many as thirty different countries, such was his fame.

And yet, today, the Natural Hygienic movement, though originally in part based in the use of cold water now rejects same, and the orthodox fraternity uses it only in a limited way under the title of hydrotherapy.

The truth of the matter is that the use of cold water is as effective today in alleviating human ills and restoring health, not to mention its value as an invigorating influence in preserving health, as it was when Priessnitz re-discovered it while watching the wounded doe immerse her wounds in the sparkling waters of the mountain torrent.

Doctor James Caleb Jackson, originator and founder of what he called the psycho-hygiene system which preceded the present natural hygiene was a dedicated "Water Cure" man, as was Russell T. Trall, who established the Hydropathic College in New York, where natural hygiene in all its phases was taught, and also Joel Shew and Isaac Jennings -- all pioneers in the hygiene or medical reform movement.

Priessnitz's work was absorbed by other systems which followed as the Kneipp and Bilz system and so on, until we find at the turn of the twentieth century an American Hydro-therapy fostered by the genius of the late John Harvey Kellogg of Battle Creek Sanitarium fame, and Dr. Simon Baruch, father of the friend of Presidents, Bernard Baruch who sometime back gave $1,000,000 for the study of Natural methods of healing. Unfortunately this money was placed at the disposal of a medically controlled board, and is being spent under medical supervision.

Nevertheless the water cure or hydropathy or what some are inclined to term hydrotherapy will live on as a monument to the little shepard lad, Vincent Priessnitz, who rediscovered the power of water as a healing agent.

Since Priessnitz's passing, the town of Grafenburg has become a shrine of the basic Nature Curists. In Grafenburg are preserved mementoes of the early days of the Grafenburg water cure where despite persecution and prosecution, the practical visionary Vincent Priessnitz plied his profession and established beyond any question the efficacy of water as a healing agent.

Among the mementoes is a letter from someone in America to Vincent Priessnitz bearing simply the address, Europe. So great had his fame grown throughout the civilized world.

To him we owe homage for his great discovery of the efficiency of cold water.

In hovel or place, cold water, even as air, heals and strengthens.

CONTENTS

A.
	Pag.
Abdominal disease	15, 40
Absorption	30
Acute diseases	15, 17
Abscesses	15, 29
Ablutions	24, *passim*
Accouchement	38
Advice, concluding	47
Ague	9
Apoplexy	21
Arthritic complaints	24
Arsenic, its ill effects	9
Asthma	7
Assimilation	16
Atony	9
Aulic council	7, 33
Austrian commission of inquiry	6

B.
Baths	12, 27
—— method of	12
Bandages, cooling	24
—— stimulating	24
Behrend, Dr., his account of the Hydropathic system	7, 8
Bleeding	17
Blindness, cures of	43, 46
Bowels, disorder of	30
—— relaxed	24
Brain, inflammation of	36, 46
Bruises	24
Burns	39

C.
Cancer	24, 35, 44
Caries	15, 24
Capillary action	22
Catarrh	38
Chest, inflammation in	36
—— complaints	24
—— pain in	40
Children	31, 43, 44
Chilblains	36
Chiragra	15
Cholera	15, 36, 45
Chronic disease	9
Claridge, Robt. Esq., his account	7
—————— his cure	32
Clothes	14, 15
Cold	29
Cold water, drinking	25, *passim*
Clyster	2
Colics	24, 39
Cold feet	36
Cotton	15
Consumption	22

	Page
Constipation	24, 39
Congestion of blood	40
—— intestine	24
Cough	38
Crises	13, 21, 28
Cure by Cold-water	41, *passim*
—— System and theory of	16
—— Practice	20
Cutaneous Functions	30, 31

D.
Deafness	30, 42, 44
Debility, general	24
Diarrhœa	21, 38
Diet	9, 11
Dinners	11
Digestion, weakness of	24, 39
Diseases, how to treat by cold water	31
—— origin of	18
Douche-bath	9, 13, 21, 29
Dress	15
Dropsy	22, 35
Drowsiness	40
Drugs, dangerous effects of	17, 26
Dysentery	15, 21
Dyspepsia	39

E.
Ear	27
—— ach	40
Efflorescent diseases	15
Engel, Dr., his account of Cold-water Cure	8
Epilepsy	38
Erysipelas	15, 36
Eruption	16
Eye bath	29
Eyes, inflammation of	21, 24, 37, 46
—— weakness of	24
—— sore	37, 38
—— pain in	37
Exercise	26, *passim*
Exhalation	30

F.
Fatigue	29
Fever	17, 33, 44, 47
—— Intermittent	7, 9, 15, 35
—— Nervous	7, 15, 35
—— Putrid	9
—— Scarlet	9
—— Phlegmatic	15
—— Inflammatory	35
Finger bath	29
Flannel	15, 33
Fomentations	24

CONTENTS

	Page
Foot baths	21, 29
Feet, cold	29
Fractures	40
Friction	22, *passim*

G.

Gastric disorders	15
Glands, tumours in	7
Gonagra	15
Graefenberg, route to	48
———— account of	8, 9
———— expenses at	9, 48
———— style of living at	12
Gripes	24, 38
Gout	7, 9, 15, 24, 31, 33, 43, 44, 46
—— in feet	15, 43
—— in hands	15, 43
—— atonic	28

H.

Half-bath	27
Head, blood to	40
———— ach	21, 40
———— cold in	38
Head bath	29
Hernia	7, 33
Heart, swelling of	8
———— inflammation of	21
Heartburn	39
Hemorrhoids	27
Hooping cough	37
Hydropathy	5, *passim*
Hypochondria	9, 15, 40
Hysterics	9, 15, 40
Hufeland, Dr.	31

I.

Jaundice	9
Indigestion	9, 39
Inflammation	15
Influenza	28, 42
Iodine, ill effects of	9
Joints, stiffness in	36, 39

L.

Leg, bath	29
Leg, sore	24, 46
Liver, swelling of	8
———— complaint	
Limbs, loss of use of	28, 33, 43
Lungs, inflammation	21

M.

Measles	7, 37, 45
Medical treatment, faults of	17
Medicine, its origin	18
Menstruation, irregularity of	41
Mercury, ill effects of, removed	9, 15
Mercurial diseases	38

N.

Nausea	41
Neck, stiff	38
Nervous affection	8
———— weakness	39
Nose	27
—— bleeding of	40

O.

Ophthalmia	37, 46

P.

	Page
Perspiration	13, *passim*
Physic	17
Piles	15, 38
Pleurisy	7, 40
Podagra	15
Priessnitz, *Vincent*, account of	6, 8
———— sagacity of	10
———— wealth of	11
———— honours to	41, 42
Prussian State inquiry	7

Q.

Quinine, its ill effects	9
Quinsy	38

R.

Respiration	19
Rheumatism	7, 15, 28, 33, 35, 43
Rickets, irregular	37
Ringworm	7, 15, 37

S.

Scarlatina	7, 37, 45
Sciatica	15, 32, 44
Scrofula	7, 9, 33
Sickness	40, 41
Sitz-bath	21, 29
Skin	21, *passim*
Sleep, loss of	40
Small-pox	7, 37
Spitting of blood from stomach	40
Spinal weakness	46
Sprains	39
Stitch, inside	40
Stomach	24
———— Debility in	39
Sweating	8, 9, 12, 18, 20, 23
Syphilis	7, 15, 38, 45

T.

Thirst	26
Throat	24
———— Sore	21, 25, 38
———— Sore inflamed	28
Tic douloureux	7, 31, 40
Tooth-ach	21, 40
Trachitis	7
Typhus	9, 42

U.

Ulcers	15
———— Syphilitic	24
———— Mercurial	38
Umschlag	24, 25
Ural complaints	24
Uterine hemorrhage	41
Vomiting	6

W.

Water	22
Weakness, general cure of	47
Wesley, Rev. John, his testimony to the efficacy of cold water	10
Wet sheet	15, 24, 25
Winter	48
Withered legs	33
Whites, the	41
Worm	37
Wounds	24, 33, 39

THE
COLD WATER CURE.

When Naaman, the Syrian, proud of the favour of his royal master, and surrounded with a glittering train of attendants, was told by the prophet, in answer to his inquiry for the means of health, to wash thrice in the waters of Jordan, his anger burst out with the indignant exclamation—" Are not Abana and Pharpar, rivers of Damascus, better than all the waters of Israel? May I not wash in *them* and be clean? So he turned, and went away in a rage." And why this anger? Whence this burst of indignation? Because, in truth, the remedy pointed out to him was simple; because, with all the pride and desire of the complicated, which pervades the heart of man, he could not, after travelling a weary journey—after vain and fruitless endeavours for health, through many years and many toils—he could not brook to be told that a remedy so rational, so simple, one which even in Damascus itself he had overlooked, should be the one, the real, the natural remedy for the disease. And so, we fear, it will be with too many of our readers, to whom we address ourselves in this humble little book, in the hope of rescuing them from the hands of surgeons and physicians and scientific charlatans, and placing them at once in possession of a true and universal remedy, which, while it ensures them health, shall cost them nothing. Let us hope, however, the words of Naaman's attendants may be fully impressed on the minds of our readers, and that like him they will have faith to try the remedy, and be healed:— " And his servants came near, and spake unto him, and said, ' My father, if the prophet had bid thee do some great thing, wouldst thou not have done it? How much rather, then, when he saith to thee, Wash and be clean?' "

Thus, then, we do not ask the British public to go on, day by day, swallowing bushels of "vegetable pills," with "fluid magnesia" to wash them down. We recommend no specific—we profess to sell them no cordial—we set before them no "balm of Gilead," nor " Balsam of Honey," nor " Life Pills," nor " Medicine without taste;" we figure to them no stethescope; nor wish to rub them till their backs are sore; no ointments, no lotions, no specifics, mineral, animal, or vegetable, are in our pharmacopœia; but we say simply to them, with the prophet Elisha, "Wash and be clean."

The remedy to which we wish to call the public attention is " *cold* water," and the system of curing diseases by it, which, for the last fifteen years, has been in active use by its peasant discoverer Vincent Priessnitz, at Grüefenberg, in Silesia, whence, under the patronage of kings and princes, it has spread over the whole of Germany; there being in every great city new institutions, under the patronage and at the expense of the Government, for the cure of diseases by the simple application of cold water alone. And first, let us back up our testimony to the virtues of the treatment of complaints by the use of cold water, with the opinion of the leading journal of Europe, which, in its critical remarks on a work recently published on Hydropathy, by R. T. Claridge, Esq., gives a short summary of the history and progress of the cold water cure and its first discoverer as follows :—

" What is hydropathy?" we expect will be the question asked by many after perusing the above title. The answer is, a system of curing all curable diseases incident to the human frame by the agency of cold spring water, air, and exercise alone. Such an allegation is startling enough, and was first received by ourselves with much distrust, living as we do in an age so fertile of imposture and pretension of mesmerism and mysticism. But we have taken pains to look into this system as practised by Vincent Priessnitz at an establishment he has founded and superintends for its application at Grüefenberg, in Austrian Silesia, and should deem ourselves negligent of our duty did we not invite public attention to the subject. If the system is fallacious, the sooner it is exposed the better; but if effective, as its advocates affirm, then will its extension confer the greatest blessing on suffering mankind. The faculty and *pharmacopolæ* will of course treat Priessnitz's pretensions with derision: but if they are well founded, and his system is generally adopted, the affair will prove no laughing matter for the doctor and the druggist, whose occupations will on such an event be clearly gone. All drugs are pronounced by Priessnitz to be poisons, and all mineral springs to contain, not life, but death, in their waters. The horse or the ox which declines Harrogate water is wiser than man; nature has made the water nauseous to warn all animals against drinking it; the animal therefore which follows instinct is right; the reasoning animal, man, is wrong. Apothecaries'-hall, our next-door neighbour, to which we have so often resorted for relief, and departed under a notion that we obtained it, now totters to a fall on the fiat of a Silesian peasant, and his name will be most bitterly cursed from Carlsbad to Cheltenham by all the lodging-house keepers of every watering-place, from Ems to Harrogate, from Toplitz to Tunbridge Wells.

Pure cold spring water is the beverage to secure health and longevity, and its application in a variety of ways, both externally and internally, is declared by Priessnitz to be " the very best of physic." Our readers may smile at our prophecy of the downfall of the druggists and the ruin of the spas; but it is, at any rate, a grave fact, if the statements now before us may be trusted, that more than 7,000 patients labouring under the most complicated forms of acute and chronic disease, many of whose cases had been resigned in despair by able physicians, have received relief under the treatment of Priessnitz at Graefenberg. But we must now introduce him and his Silesian establishment more formally to our readers.

Vincent Priessnitz is the son of a small farmer, and was born on the land upon which his present establishment is placed. His father's humble means prevented Vincent from obtaining more than a very limited education, and the father's blindness in advanced life cast the management of the farm upon the son. In the immediate neighbourhood there lived an old man who used to practise the water cure upon cattle, and it is supposed that from this source the young Priessnitz derived his first ideas of the subject. His first patient seems to have been himself, and rather marvellous is the narrative of the events given by Mr. Claridge, whose words we will quote.

"Early in life, whilst engaged in hay-making, an accident which befel him was the principal cause of the dispensation of one of the greatest blessings to suffering humanity; he was kicked in the face by a horse, which knocked him down, and the cart passing over his body broke two of his ribs. A surgeon from Freiwaldau being called in, declared that he never could be so cured as to be fit for work again. Having always possessed great presence of mind, and an unusual degree of firmness, the young Priessnitz not being pleased with this prognostication of the doctor, and being somewhat acquainted already with the treatment of trifling wounds by the means of cold water, determined to endeavour to cure himself. To effect this, his first care was to replace his ribs, and this he did by leaning his abdomen with all his might against a table or a chair, and holding his breath so as to swell out his chest. This painful operation was attended with the success he expected; the ribs being thus replaced, he applied wet cloths to the parts affected, drank plentifully of water, ate sparingly, and remained in perfect repose. In ten days he was able to go out, and at the end of a year he was again at his occupation in the fields."

The Silesian surgeon's notion that a couple of broken ribs would disable a peasant boy for life, does not indicate much medical skill on his part; but if the above narrative is accurate, the facts disclose in the young Priessnitz those qualities of sagacity, firmness, self-possession, and patience, which are so essential for the constitution of the high medical character. The fame of Priessnitz's extraordinary cure soon spread around the neighbourhood, and brought patients begging his assistance and advice. He shortly became so famous that the envy of the medical practitioners was awakened, and they denounced him to the authorities at Vienna as a dangerous empiric, whose quackery should be stopped by the strong arm of the law. Be it known that in arbitrary Austria quacks are not permitted to mangle and poison the Emperor's subjects *à discretion*, to their own appetite's content, as in free England. Happy Austria! It was alleged that the sponges and wet cloths which Priessnitz employed in the ablution of his patients were medicated with drugs more potent than pure spring water. Upon this denunciation Aulic inspectors came to Graefenberg to investigate; the sponges were decomposed, and nothing either worse or better than water was detected in their contents. After a searching examination, the commission appointed by the Austrian government to inquire found that the only agents employed by Priessnitz in effecting his cures were pure cold water, air, and exercise, and were so convinced of the benefits derivable from his system, and its perfect safety to patients in the most advanced stages of disease, that on their report the most jealous government in Europe allowed Priessnitz to continue his operations. Those who came to punish remained to praise, and since that time the hydropathist has been honoured by the friendship of many members of the Imperial Family, and by distinguished individuals from every quarter of the continent. In England the name of Priessnitz has only just been heard, and, in the list of his patients for 1840 only two Englishmen are found, whereas there are 367 Austrians (the prophet *has* honour in his own country), and no fewer than 527 from Prussia. One of the English patients, we presume is Mr. Claridge, the compiler of the work before us, the materials of which he informs his readers were gathered from the writings of many German authors, medical and otherwise, who, after experiencing the benefits of Priessnitz's treatment in their own persons, or witnessing its salutary effects upon others, felt themselves bound to publish his merits to the world. Mr. Claridge, who sought a remedy for tic-douloureux, and found it at Graefenberg, avows himself to be influenced by the same amiable and candid motives, and is therefore entitled to be treated with respect, however "doctors may differ" in their estimate of the system he so warmly praises.

"On the day of our departure," writes Mr. Claridge, "we had been at Graefenberg three months, during which time our health was perfectly established; we acquired the habit of living more moderately, of taking more exercise, of drinking more water, and of using it more freely in external ablutions than we were accustomed to; and I may add, that we have learned how to allay pain, how to ward off disease, and, I hope, how to preserve health. My sojourn at Graefenberg will ever be matter of self-congratulation to me, and will be amongst my happiest recollections. If I am instrumental in relieving the sufferings of my countrymen, if I succeed in bringing to their notice a system calculated to be of such essential benefit to them, if I can prevail upon them to participate in the happy effects of the treatment which I have myself experienced, my feelings of satisfaction, arising from my residence at Graefenberg, will be heightened in no ordinary degree."

Mr. Claridge gives the following account of the hydropathic treatment to which he himself was subjected :—

"Having at last made up my mind to become one of Priessnitz's patients, I was prepared for his coming in the morning. The first thing he did was to request me to strip and go into the large cold bath, where I remained two or three minutes. On coming out he gave me instructions, which I pursued as follows :—At 4 o'clock in the morning my servant folded me in a large blanket, over which he placed as many things as I could conveniently bear, so that no external air could penetrate. After perspiration commenced it was allowed to continue for an hour; he then brought a pair of straw shoes, wound the blanket close about my body, and in this state of perspiration I descended to a large cold bath, in which I remained three minutes, then dressed, and walked until breakfast, which was composed of milk, bread, butter, and strawberries (the wild strawberry in this country grows in abundance from the latter end of May until late in October). At ten o'clock I proceeded to the douche, under which I remained four minutes, returned home, and took a sitz and foot-bath, each for 15 minutes; dined at 1 o'clock."

We may observe parenthetically that the dinners at Gräefenberg are of a plentiful but coarse description; the usual alternations of the greasy and the sour met with at German *tables d'hôte* must be encountered there. It appears that M. Priessnitz permits his patients to eat at dinner what and as much as they please; but while under his care they must drink only water.

"At 4 proceeded again to the douche; at 7 repeated the sitz and foot-baths; retired to bed at half-past 9, previously having my feet and legs bound up in cold wet bandages. I continued this treatment for three months, and during that time walked about 1,000 miles. Whilst thus subjected to the treatment I enjoyed more robust health than I had ever done before; the only visible effect that I experienced was an eruption on both my legs, but which, on account of the bandages, produced no pain. It is to these bandages, the perspiration, and the baths, that I am indebted for the total departure of my rheumatism."

The above is one specimen of hydropathic treatment; but a great variety of modes may be found in the volume, to which we refer those readers who desire fuller information on the subject. All these dressings and undressings, washings and rubbings, and bandages, this perpetual buttoning and unbuttoning, must be terribly irksome, but the fact of so many submitting to their infliction strongly indicates that benefits have been felt to flow from Priessnitz's operations, else would the irritable invalids, whom luxurious living had debilitated, never have endured it for a single week. Mr. Claridge enumerates the diseases which are curable by the Hydropathic process, and among them may be found some of the most frequent and many of the most formidable which attack the human frame. Several cases of patients are given, but we have not space to recite them; we will, however, make an extract from a letter of Dr. Behrend, of Berlin, unfolding his views of Priessnitz's proceedings. We have no ground for suspecting any bias in favour of Priessnitz's plans to exist in the mind of the Prussian physician, whom we should rather surmise to be disdainful of the Silesian peasant, yet Dr. Behrend thus delivers his opinions:—

"The new method of applying cold water in the cure of most diseases, internally and externally, was discovered by a peasant named Priessnitz, a man endowed with superior intelligence and extraordinary penetration. It has been in use for eight years, with the consent of the Austrian Government, at Gräefenberg, a village in Austrian Silesia. So many cures have been effected by this peasant, and cures of so astonishing a nature, that numbers of patients have arrived not only from Germany but other countries; and doctors, who prefer instructing themselves to blindly opposing so new and wonderful a discovery, are on the increase. The number of patients of all ranks of society during this year was more than 1,500 (not including 50 doctors). The village of Gräefenberg is already changed into a small town. The matter has been scrupulously examined by the Prussian Government, which has confirmed the happy results arising from this new application of cold water. The method is named Hydriatique, or Hydropathy, and has attracted the attention of all the Governments of Germany. The great success which Priessnitz has obtained, and still obtains every day, does not depend upon the quality or composition of the water, which is pure spring water, but on the new manner in which it is administered.

"Establishments have been already formed of the same nature at Breslaw, Brunswick, Dresden, Gotha, Bavaria, Cassell, &c.; there are two at Berlin, and a friend of mine is on the point of establishing one in some town or village of Belgium. After having seen such extraordinary success obtained by this hydriatic method—after having examined, without prejudice, the persons returning cured from Gräefenberg, many of whom were connexions of my own, I went there with two other professional men in order to see with our own eyes. We stayed there six weeks, strictly examining the peasant Priessnitz's method.

"Practitioner as I am, of fifteen years' standing, and editor for six years of a medical journal, I was at first a little mistrustful of this novelty, and compared it with many others whose authors pretended to reform the medical art, and who have completely vanished. But that which I saw with my own eyes at Gräefenberg and other similar establishments struck me, as it will you, with astonishment. I have seen asthmas and pleurisies completely cured in three or four days by cold water only. I have seen an old intermittent fever cured by cold water, without quinine or any other remedy than cold water. I have seen measles, scarlatina, small-pox, nervous fevers, rheumatism, scrofula, hernia, trachitis or complaints of the throat, gout, ringworm, syphilis, tic-douloureux, and other nervous affections; tumours in the glands, swelling of the heart, liver, and all effects of mercury, and many other diseases, cured by simple cold water, without the aid of any other remedy whatever; and in a comparatively shorter time and a more favourable manner for the constitution, than could have been attained by any other means. Cold water is administered in all diseases, internally and externally, but the method of application is varied according to the individual and the case. Cold water serves sometimes as a revulsive and sometimes as a depressive agen, and in all these cases the efficacy of water is so clearly manifested that to doubt is impossible."*

* See also the following testimonial, in a letter written to the editor of the *Gazette Médicale de Paris*, 13th Jan. 1840, by Dr. Engel of Vienna:—

Sir—In visiting your capital, the centre of civilisation, it is impossible for a foreigner, animated with the desire of instruction, not to make every effort to profit by the perfection which Arts and Sciences have attained there. Whatever may be his studies, it is certain that he will add greatly to his previous knowledge and information; in the midst of his admiration he will, notwithstanding, be astonished to find a total ignorance in this civilised country of the progress in a branch of the medical art which has succeeded to such an extraordinary extent in Germany. Excited by a legitimate national pride, and by a consciousness of duty which he is bound as a medical man to perform, he feels the necessity of making known this valuable discovery, of the efficacy of which, from the numerous experiments that have been made, there can exist no doubt.

These are the motives, Sir, which led me to forward these lines to you, and to beg, if you think them calculated to be useful, that you will insert them in your valuable journal.

The narrow limits to which I am obliged to confine myself will not permit me to treat this important subject, so as to make you comprehend entirely hydropathy, or the cold water cure. I will only, for the present moment, give the leading features of the system, saying something of its origin and progress, in order to attract the attention of the French medical profession to the subject. If, as I venture to hope, these lines are favourably received, I propose afterwards publishing a small work, more in detail, developing the theory and practice of a treatment (the astonishing efficacy of which I have proved myself), by enumerating many facts chosen out of a great number, all of which came under my own especial observation.

In all ages water has been employed in different cases. I believe, however, that our times are destined to see the use of it much more extended, and to show us in what manner medical science, now so complicated, had its origin. In fact, it is not from any profound researches, it is not by the learned availing themselves of the knowledge of their predecessors that this powerful, though simple, method, of curing disease has been discovered. It is to a plain countryman, guided by his observations of nature, that humanity is indebted.

Priessnitz, whose name is celebrated throughout Germany, inhabits Gräefenberg, a hamlet until a recent period completely isolated and unknown, upon a mountain of the chain of the Sudates, on the frontier of the Austrian monarchy. In his retired retreat, deprived of all medical aid, he attempted to cure the diseases by which he and his relations were afflicted: encouraged by success, he next endeavoured to cure persons attacked by the gout, which defies all other remedies, and which is an endemic in this country. He again succeeded. His observations were increased, his judgment strengthened, and his quick perceptions confirmed. The fame of his cures became known, his renown brought invalids not only from all parts of Austria, but also from distant countries; almost all returned convalescent, or relieved more effectually than could ever have been expected. But now a greater triumph awaited nature's doctor. After having suffered all sorts of calumny, of envy, and contempt from scientific conceit, he at last saw his efforts appreciated; all are now ready to do him justice, to follow him in his practice. Many considerable establishments have been created upon the model of that which he founded; and Hydropathy is honoured and respected throughout all Germany.

As I have already said, it was on a high mountain that Priessnitz first commenced his cures; there are now about two hundred and fifty invalids at this place. It was in the middle of a forest that he thus undertook the cure, without any other auxiliaries than pure air and water, springing from the rocks, and a wonderful talent to adapt and modify the treatment requisite for all; no two persons being treated exactly alike in this apparently simple and uniform cure.

But it is useless to ask him the theory or the principles of his treatment; however active and energetic may be his ideas, he cannot express them; it is only by closely observing his actions that you can form any idea of the manner in which he follows the laws of physic and physiology, the names of which sciences are unknown to him.

In this wild situation you see scattered several peasants' cottages, and also Priessnitz's house, which has nothing to distinguish it from the others. Amongst these cottages are two large buildings, constructed principally of wood, destined to lodge those who have come to consult him. Though the rooms are small and uncomfortable, his patients, however, far from being disheartened, are all sustained by the hope of recovering their health. Many remain during winter, which is extremely severe in these mountains, where in the month of August I have found, before the rising of the sun, but 6° of heat, Reaumur (45° Fahrenheit). But Priessnitz thinks the lower the temperature of the water is, the more efficacious it will prove. The cure once commenced cannot be discontinued without injury to the patient.

I shall now enter into some details of the way an invalid employs his time at Gräefenberg, which will at the same time give an idea of the general treatment. I say idea, because Priessnitz varies it in so many ways according to the persons to whom it is applied, that you must have witnessed the treatment to judge of the variety of its applications. That which distinguishes this, however, from every other cure, is the absence of all pharmaceutic agency; it is the perspiration and the crisis that characterise it, and which remove all the diseases submitted to the action of cold water.

The invalid is awoke at four or five o'clock in the morning, then enveloped almost hermetically in a thick, coarse, woollen blanket, the head only is left uncovered, by which all contact with the exterior air is carefully avoided. Presently the heat accumulates round the invalid, depending upon the heat of the atmosphere, and he perspires sufficiently to wet the whole of the coverings; during this time he may drink as much cold water as he pleases. After he has thus sweated the allotted time, he takes a cold bath. The first impression is doubtless disagreeable; but once overcome, an agreeable sensation follows, as the pores dilated by the heat absorb the liquid.

After much observation it is found to be the moment when that salutary exchange takes place which purifies the system. This sudden variation of temperature never has produced any serious accident; all irritation produced by stimulants is carefully avoided, the lungs are not heated by breathing hot air, as in the Russian baths, the skin only being slightly stimulated. On coming

All this sounds marvellous and incredible, and will be long before it wins English belief; but Dr. Behrend is an experienced medical practitioner, who went to see and examine for himself, and he informs us that both the Austrian and Prussian Governments are satisfied of the validity of Priessnitz's alleged powers of healing. Would it not be well worth the while of some intelligent and enterprising young English medical practitioner, many of which class now find it so hard to obtain employment, to spend a few months at Gräefenberg, and thoroughly study Priessnitz's system? The name of Gräefenberg is so little familiar to the English reader, and the place itself lies so wide of the ordinary travelling track, that we will point out its site. It is situated half way up one of the mountains of the Sudates, in Silesia, 260 miles from Berlin, 200 from Dresden, and 175 from Vienna. A traveller from England may proceed thither either by way of the Rhine, Frankfort, Leipsic, and Dresden, or by Hamburgh and Berlin, thanks to steam-boats and railways, at an outlay not exceeding £10, provisions excluded. Living at Gräefenberg, which, be it noted, is so destitute of comfort that no one can be suspected of lingering there for caprice or amusement, as at Wiesbaden, or any other fashionable spa—living is so cheap, that board, lodging, and medical attendance may be obtained for £1 per week. It would not, therefore, out of the bath the invalid is dried and quickly dressed; if able, he then takes a walk, during which he drinks abundantly of cold water.

He ought, however, to avoid excess, which is manifested by a disagreeable weight of the stomach. Habit does wonders in this respect. You see persons almost hydrophobic at the commencement, who, after a time, drink from twenty to thirty glasses of water a day.

Breakfast consists of bread, cold milk, and fruit. Priessnitz considers all heated things to be prejudicial and debilitating to the stomach; and this opinion is confirmed by his experiments upon animals. After breakfast, every one is expected to take a long walk, and then to proceed to the douche, leaving a sufficient interval to avoid accidents.

Invalids, whose skins are habitually cold, dry, and hard, will perspire more easily from cold ablutions; those who suffer from local complaints, are relieved by more or less frequent fomentations; those who are attacked by chronic evils, which are more obstinate, are submitted to the influence of cold water.

I have already made mention of the douche; it is very interesting to observe the efficacy of this last manner of applying cold water. A gouty subject, for instance, who submits his hands and feet, or any swelled part, to the action of a strong fall of water, experiences the following phenomenon: his skin becomes quite red, and he then feels an intolerable itching, occasioned either by re-absorption, or oftener by a topical suppuration.

Invalids should generally drink much cold water, and take a great deal of exercise if they can support fatigue. The dinner hour is one o'clock. I think it would be difficult to see a more extraordinary appetite than that possessed by Priessnitz's invalids, who all dine in the same room.

Individuals afflicted by chronic diseases, whose digestion has been deranged by a number of remedies, are not long before they re-establish its functions, by the return of their vital force. The food is plain and abundant; the only objection to it is, that the dishes are sometimes too coarse for delicate stomachs. Each person eats as much as he pleases, or according to his appetite.

If the weakness of the patients, or the crisis already begun does not prevent it, they recommence some hours after dinner the treatment of the morning; the douche is, however, forbidden, as too irritating. After a slight supper of cold milk and bread, every one retires to rest. The occupations of the day are a guarantee for repose during the night.

The sensation caused by the Hydropathic treatment differs essentially from that arising from any other method of curing.

In the beginning, the return of strength and the awakening of the torpid faculties are agreeably felt; excitement is not limited to the affected organs, but becomes general, and produces a salutary revolution in all the vital powers.

The true febrile symptoms develop themselves; the pains already existing, become more intense: old diseases, in appearance cured long since, re-appear: these effects are but the forerunners of a more determined crisis.

Almost all the patients who have followed this treatment for some time, feel an itching and a sharp pain in the skin, which is sometimes covered with spots or pimples of different forms.

The diseases which are caused by the irregularity of the nervous functions, are generally limited to this sort of crisis. If we, on the contrary, treat of the cure of what are called material diseases, the phenomena which they manifest are sufficient to convince the most incredulous of the efficacy of this treatment. The sweating, more abundant every day, contains morbid matter, the nature of which differs according to the disease. The different shades of the viscosity and of the odours, prove this most incontestably. The number of abscesses which make their appearance sooner or later, under the influence of cold water, purify the system of corrupt humours. Whilst the invalids are thus covered with abscesses, an abundant secretion is discharged by perspiration, the urine, or the urethra. They then find themselves physically and morally better, their appetites increase, their pains are diminished, and, finally, their health is established.

I shall finish this notice by enumerating the diseases which more especially are cured or relieved by cold water, and examples of which are found in great numbers in the Hydropathic establishments.

I may fairly hope, as this method becomes better known and more practised, under various circumstances, and in different climates, that it will be more and more appreciated; my observations have convinced me that the mode of treatment is efficacious, principally in chronic diseases, accompanied by atony; in all nervous affections, spasms, pains of which medicine will not discover the cause; in cases of obstructions of the stomach, and all the systematic evils which arise from them; such as indigestion, hypochondria, piles, jaundice, &c. Also in cases of gout, rheumatism, scrofula; diseases affecting women, such as hysterics, &c. In fact, cold water is perfectly successful in a number of diseases, beyond the reach of medicine altogether. I have again had occasion to admire the result of the application of cold water in cases of ague, accompanied by symptoms of fever, such as nervous, typhus, putrid and scarlet fevers; but its most signal triumphs are obtained over those serious derangements of the system produced by the abuse of drugs, such as when the passage of the system is obstructed by quinine; or when consumptions are produced by iodine, arsenic, or the consequences of mercury, tartar emetic, and other dangerous medicaments, have manifested themselves.

be a costly experiment for a student to make, and if the system to which we direct his attention can effect a tithe of the wonders attributed to it, an English practitioner would derive both fame and fortune from his trip.

The main difficulty to be overcome by a student we suspect to be Priessnitz's inability to communicate his method of distinguishing diseases and applying the appropriate remedies. It is true he employs only one agent—water; but then he applies it in an almost infinite variety of ways, and is said to treat no two cases precisely alike. From his deficient education, and also, now, from the complete occupation of his time, it is quite hopeless that Priessnitz can transmit his knowledge to posterity by his pen. Disciples, therefore, must gather wisdom from his lips, or rather from a minute observation of his every act; for he is a man of few words, and retains all the simplicity of his early peasant life. His sagacity in detecting the very seat of disease is little short of the miraculous, if all we have read of him be true; but, allowing for the exaggeration of admirers, and he himself, simple man, is quite innocent of advertisement or puff, it must be very extraordinary. We hear that none of the establishments set up in imitation of him have as yet equalled their model. We should, therefore, advise a still more strict analysis of the Gräefenberg waters, to ascertain whether they may not be mineral after all. It is confidently affirmed that no water can be more free from any mineral admixture or taint, as Priessnitz would call it, than that used at Gräefenberg—but let this point be put beyond all doubt. Priessnitz's honesty seems equal to his skill. He does not pretend to the possession of a panacea—he at once tells a patient whether he can cure him or not, and frequently rejects applications. Neither does he profess to restore the powers of nature, if extinguished by disease or a long course of irregular living. He says he can cure all curable diseases, and refresh powers impaired to a degree which many physicians would pronounce desperate.

It is no part of the task which we have prescribed ourselves in noticing the volume before us to advocate M. Priessnitz's system, nor can we go in our belief of its efficacy to the extent of his enthusiastic Continental eulogists; but it certainly deserves investigation in this country, where, until very recently, its existence even was unknown. To speak of cold pure spring water as a medicine is, we are well aware, at once to raise a laugh or provoke a sneer, especially in this country, where a horror almost of cold water prevails. With rare exceptions, among the refined, a majority of even decent English men and women content themselves with washing their hands and faces twice a-day in cold water, and their feet once a week in warm.* All the other portions of the skin, which has such important functions to discharge in our animal economy, is left neglected. The nations of antiquity, with one common consent, used baths and ablutions of the whole person. The Spartans strung their nerves for Thermopylæ by a daily bath in the Eurotas; and among the Romans the current proverb, ' *Nec degere nec natare didicet*,' shows how habitual was the use of water with them. If we direct our observation to a modern nation, the Turks, we may perceive the benefits derivable from daily ablutions. Indigestion is but little known among the Turks, and yet no people on earth do more to induce it. On one day a Turk will dine on cucumber and cheese, the next he will gorge himself from a dozen greasy dishes; for three months together he will be twelve hours a-day on horseback, and for the ensuing three months he will, perhaps, scarcely stir from his sofa, and yet it is rare to meet a dyspeptic Turk. With such habits, how can we account for this fact? We attribute the Turk's exemption from dyspepsia to the daily ablution which his religion prescribes.

But the direct application of cold water to the cure of diseases is not so great a novelty as some of Priessnitz's admirers appear to imagine. Hippocrates, the father of medicine, prescribes cold water for the treatment of the most serious diseases; Celsus and Galen recommend its use both in sickness and health, and we could give a long list of writers who have adopted the same views. We may mention that nearly a century ago, in 1747, John Wesley published a book entitled *Primitive Physic, or an Easy and Natural Method of Curing most Diseases*, in which he gives his opinion that water, properly applied, will cure almost every disease which flesh is heir to. The founder of Methodism was not a physician, but he was a shrewd observer, and the valuable little work to which we have alluded is full of excellent advice, of which a regular practitioner need not be ashamed. But simple remedies do not suit this luxurious generation; they long for what is elaborate and costly; they are willing to " do some great thing;" but when merely told to " wash and be clean," like Naaman the Syrian, they turn away from the river in a rage.

Such are the opinions of the editor of the *Times*, and we can add but little to the brief account there given of the inventor, M. Priessnitz, or of his establishment at Gräefenberg, unless in translating from the work of a celebrated German physician the following narrative of his visit to Gräefenberg, with an account of his treatment and cure. After relating the particulars of his journey, he says:—" I soon had an interview with this wonder of the healing art, and proved that his portraits much belied him,

* There is an American story which bears upon this editorial observation.—A lady, whose child was pining, took it to a celebrated physician:—" Sir, my child is very ill." " Yes, Madam, I perceive it looks very ill." " What shall I do, Sir? would you recommend me to take it to the springs?" " By all means, Madam; take it to the springs—lose no time in taking it to the springs." " Shall I go to Saratoga, Sir? what springs would you recommend?" " Any springs, Madam, where there is plenty of soap and water."

for while he was neither so handsome, or so witty, as they made him seem, there was a marked expression of calmness, goodness and reflective power in the countenance of Vincent Priessnitz. He introduced his fair and good-looking wife; she is very clever, and natural in manners, and manages the domestic economy of this large household with great housewife skill.

"I had used the caution, indispensable to all who visit Gräefenberg, of sending a letter to Priessnitz beforehand, to secure accommodation, and even then had much difficulty in obtaining it. Since my visit, however, I learn that an immense building has been erected, and that there is no longer difficulty in lodging the numerous aspirants after health. The furniture of my room was a wooden bedstead, a mattress of straw, a thin feather bed and sheet, a large feather bed in place of blankets to cover me, and two pillows; a chest of drawers, a small table, and two chairs of common wood, shape and workmanship; a boot-jack, a bottle, two glasses, and an enormous wash-hand basin. Those who cannot do without mattresses must hire them at Freiwaldau, about three-quarters of a mile from Gräefenberg. Just as I had got my things to rights, a bell rang, and announced the dinner hour at Priessnitz's large establishment. On entering the dining room, a noble saloon in the building, of colossal dimensions, I was surprised at the number of persons assembled (upwards of two hundred), and sitting together, without distinction of rank or age, at long tables placed in lines. At the centre table M. Priessnitz himself presides; indeed he is always present at every meal—breakfast, dinner, or supper. Here he holds, as it were, his public audiences, and is consulted by his patients, some of whom have always some questions to ask him, which they do aloud, and without any restraint. To hear the laughing and sounds of merriment you would hardly fancy yourself amongst a band of invalids. Now came on the dinner—soup and something fried was first served—then boiled beef with sharp sauce, pickled cucumbers, and minced meat with green peas. Vegetables are scarce at these dinners, but not prohibited—cabbages, however, and sour crout were plentiful. Mutton, veal and pork, alternately with fowls, roast ducks, salads, preserves and pastry of all kinds, made up the repast. Fresh butter served as a dessert. The bread is brown, but white may be purchased, if preferred. Fruits *in season* may be eaten, but these are not included in the charge for board. Every one drinks at table large quantities of cold water—each from about twenty to thirty glasses a day. Priessnitz advises his patients to drink copiously of cold water, both as a remedy to repair the loss of liquid by strong perspiration every day, and to assist in the dissolution and excretory evacuation of morbid matters. Hence the servants are busily engaged in running backwards and forwards, and filling the bottles with excellent cold water, from a fountain which springs just two steps from the dining room—where, morning and evening, you may see standing round a circle of merry, laughing invalids, who now and then amuse themselves by wagering who can drink most.

"And here I was much struck with the quantity of food consumed by the invalids under the eye of their physician. As all his treatment tends to give activity and vigour to the system, Priessnitz, it seems, far from lowering the system by severe diet or diminution of food, permits them to eat what and as much as they please, except foreign spices and spirituous liquors, which are strictly prohibited. He gives them food plain, solid, and coarse; and thus the patients acquire confidence, for they soon find that they eat more, and with better appetites, than ever they did in their lives before; and digest, as invalids, meats and other matters, which, in health, at the best of times, they would not have ventured upon. In short, instead of invalids, you would think, to see the company at Gräefenberg eat, that they were a number of hungry workmen, hard-working, robust, and healthy.

"After dinner I took an opportunity to consult Priessnitz [*] on my own case. I told him that I had tried his system, and cured myself of all my other ailments but a chronic cold in the head, which I could not get rid of, and which gave me a great deal of annoyance. He gave his opinion that the cold-water treatment (the sweating, particularly, and the bath to follow), would restore me, and recommended a preparatory bath; and told me to let my landlord know. Every peasant at Gräefenberg who has

---

[*] On the 4th of October, 1841, he attained his forty-second year; but from the causes we have stated, he appears somewhat older. Notwithstanding his astounding success, his accumulation of wealth (of which he is now said to possess upwards of £50,000), and the manner in which he is courted and respected by the first nobles in Germany, M. Priessnitz retains all the humility of his former humble station. It is the custom in this country, with the peasantry, to kiss the hands of their superiors, on entering and leaving a room. *If ladies are present he never omits doing this.* He is a man of deep reflection, and of few words, for he *says but little,* and rarely promises any thing; consequently, his words, when spoken, are considered as sacred by high and low as the responses of the Delphic Oracle. Many people complain that he does not talk enough; and *doctors* who come here to learn the treatment, say that he *never explains anything to them.* With respect to the first allegation, it must be evident, that a man who has all the year round from 500 to 600 patients, besides the peasantry of the neighbourhood that may require his aid, cannot have a great deal of breath to throw away. Let any person speak to him on his own or his family's case, and he will find his reply that of a man of profound sense,—a reply that he, Priessnitz, never wishes to retract, and for which he will give his reasons in the most unaffected manner possible. But with respect to the second complaint, it must be avowed that he has no very great regard for medical men, because no one has suffered more from *their vindictive feelings* than himself; besides, he has ever found it a work of supererogation to endeavour to dispossess them of their prejudices; nor has he time or inclination to enter into disputes upon a mode of treatment which he knows, as directly emanating from nature, to be always true to itself.—*Claridge on Hydropathy.*

a house, lets off all the rooms he can spare to patients who cannot find room at Priessnitz's establishment. Every house, therefore, has a room fitted up for the baths, with all the necessary apparatus: there is also, near each house, a spring of water, which is conveyed by pipes into this room. Used to the method of treatment, the landlord himself generally acts as bath servant for the men, and the landlady for females. To come to my preparatory bath :—

" I had first to strip myself to the skin, and then the bath servant (my landlord) wrapped a cloak round me, and gave me a pair of straw slippers. Thus accoutred, I walked to a small bath-room, where I entered a bath, in which there was water to the depth of a few inches only, at a temperature of 61° Fahrenheit. After being washed and rubbed over many times from head to foot, I returned back to my room well dried and rubbed, and after dressing myself went and took a pleasant walk for exercise in the open air. All new comers are ordered to take these preparatory baths for a longer or shorter time, according to the nature of their complaint, or the degree of susceptibility, previous to Priessnitz's permitting them to plunge into the cold bath. Indeed, in some cases, the patient is compelled during the whole time of his cure to confine himself to these baths.

" The bell for supper rang at seven. This meal, like the breakfast, is made of cold milk, brown bread, and fresh butter. Before going to rest the patients spend two or three hours together in the saloon, and these are the pleasantest of the day. Some smoke (in the billiard-room); others chat and play (but *not* at cards); sometimes there is a dance, sometimes singing, for music is always in attendance. In the evening, too, arrives the messenger who brings letters and news from home, and who carries away also those that we have written. Tired with travelling, I soon took my leave and retired to my bed, where, notwithstanding its hardness, I slept soundly. At four o'clock in the morning my bath-man aroused me, and proceeded to pack me up in the usual manner for the sweating process. I was turned out of bed, and he took off a sheet and a wadded counterpane, which Priessnitz had sent me (as I was not in the habit of sleeping between two feather beds, according to the custom in this part of the country), and then he placed on the bed a large blanket, on which I laid myself quite naked. Now began the packing up, and soon my very handy host had wrapped me so tight and so close that I could not move or stir. Over the blanket the featherbed was placed, and upon that the wadded counterpane, and over all these my cloak. These he well tucked up, so that I looked like a mummy in its swathing folds; and then to finish his job, he buried my head deep down in pillows, so that I was all covered but my eyes, nose, and mouth. The head, it seems, however, is not always covered, but only at the desire of Priessnitz or the request of the patient himself. ' I hope you will soon sweat, Sir,' said the bath-man on leaving me, and in furtherance of this friendly wish, came back to me every now and then to see how I was getting on. I did not at all relish the operation; as how should I, rolled up in a coarse woollen blanket, the long hair of which tickled and irritated my skin, and without being able to move? I felt it very disagreeable and uncomfortable. I dropped off to sleep in a short time, which I afterwards learnt is not a good thing; and as the temperament of my system was rather dry than moist, I had to lay two hours in this awkward position, until the sweat came on by very concentration of the perspiration, and the heat showed itself on the skin. In most patients this process occupies less time, but it depends of course on the temperament of the patient. As soon as my bath-man saw I was in a state of perspiration, he threw open the windows, and gave me every now and then cold water to drink. The intention of both is to refresh the lungs by the inhalation of fresh air, so cheering and reviving the strength of the body, and preserving it from the languid weakness ensuing from the heat. The drinking cold water when the perspiration is on, renders the respiratory organs more active; whilst to drink it before the perspiration had broken out would check it. After perspiring two hours, thus enduring four hours of this unpleasant situation, Priessnitz came in and released me by saying that I had sweated enough. This perspiration, it appears, should never be allowed to go until weakness is felt; it lasts generally from half an hour to two hours from the time of its commencement. The bath-man then closed the window, and released my head from its pillowy grave, and quickly divested me of all the envelopes except the blanket, which he loosened just enough to withdraw the urinal which he had placed in the bed; he then put on my feet the straw slippers. Priessnitz then directed me to be seated and hold out my hands, which he wetted frequently with cold water, and handed me the basin, telling me to wash my face. I then got up from the bed, wrapped in the blanket, and still reeking with perspiration. My step was light and free, and I felt neither weakness nor inconvenience, and walked down the stairs and out of the house to the bath-room. Priessnitz went before, I followed in the centre, and behind me was the bath-man bearing the sheet and cloak. After I had washed my hands and face and thrown off the blanket, Priessnitz directed me to go into the preparatory bath of tepid water, in which I was well washed and rubbed, as on the day before; I then for an instant plunged into a cold-bath, the water of which runs through the bath, coming in fresh on one side and going out at the other. I next got back to my preparatory bath as quickly as I could, whence, after another good rubbing, I plunged several times into the cold bath, rubbing my limbs well after each plunge, and then came back as a finale to the tepid bath, where I did not long remain, going back to my room, and was rubbed and dried. I then put on my clothes and went out for a walk. I felt all over in a delightful glow, and a remarkable strength both of mind and body. In the evening I again had to go through this sweating process, with the addition of a similar course of baths; but omitting the preparatory bath, I on the next day plunged at once into the cold bath on coming out of bed, first, however, washing my hands and neck, a necessary precaution which should always be rigidly observed. This cold bath shocks at first, but it will be less felt if the patient, instead of tardily and slowly approaching his danger, were to plunge into his fate at once. I advise all patients to hold their breath and plunge right in, so as to let the water cover even the head, then rub well, as long as they can, the diseased parts with the hand, and keep in about from half a minute to five, according to Priessnitz's directions, but never more unless specially ordered. The patient should not stand or lie still in the bath. This is a mischievous error—jump and kick about, rub yourself as much as possible, and the shivering sensation will not trouble you."

(The worthy doctor then goes largely into the question of perspiration, which we have fully discussed in a subsequent part of our work.) "As I had resolved to make myself acquainted with and experimentalise with, on my own body, all the processes of which the Hydropathic system is composed, I soon got permission from Priessnitz to go to the douche, though he enjoined me to use it only in moderation, and leave it off as soon as I felt any irritation from it. The number of douches at Gräefenberg is ten; two near the houses at the foot of the hill on which the village stands are not of great consequence. They are only used when the weather is too rough to enable the patients to mount the hill, where are the higher ones secluded in a forest, and at least three-quarters of a mile from Gräefenberg; two of the highest are set apart exclusively for the use of the ladies. The water springing from thence is the lowest in temperature and falls in a column an inch and a half in diameter, from a height of twelve to fifteen feet. The water running down from them is led by spouts, and forms six other douches for the use of the male patients; these six douches are raised one above another, the water falls from twelve to twenty feet, and the temperature varies from 0° to 10° Reaumur, depending on the time of year and hour of the day.

"The morning is the right time for the douche. After dinner, it is not advisable to take it. If heated with walking, we waited until we were a little cooled; but the douche must not be taken when the patient feels cold. The hands, face, and chest must be wetted well over, before exposing the body to the action of the douche; and the water should be caught at first in the hands, held over the head, so that the whole body may have a good wetting all over, previous to commencing the local action on the diseased part. The nape of the neck, back, stomach, and thighs, are the parts to be exposed to the column of water; not so the head or chest. I was instructed to move about, and rub, or be rubbed, as much as possible during the time I was en douche, bringing the water to bear as much as possible on the diseased part. At first, the douche is taken for two minutes only; afterwards, it is extended, but gradually, even to fifteen minutes. When I left the bath, in common with the other patients, I was dried, and dressed myself as quickly as I could, and set off in a brisk walk to keep off any feeling of cold, which too often comes on from remaining too long at the douche. Some patients there are, who have taken the douche from thirty to forty minutes, but this is foolish bravado, like an excess in the perspiration or drinking. The cure is made no faster by such means; on the contrary, is frequently retarded by them. Those, therefore, who go to Gräefenberg to be cured, should abide implicitly by Priessnitz's directions as to the time and manner of sweating, the duration of the preparatory baths, the parts to be exposed to the action of the douche, the quantity of water to be taken internally, and the nature of the bandages to be applied. As respects the effects of the cold-water treatment, it depends quite as much on the period when the disease shows itself, as upon the manner in which it appears, or the alterations it produces in the system, and the nature of the disease, and the physical peculiarities of the invalid.

"At the first part of our stay at Gräefenberg, the mind is pleasantly and agreeably impressed. Air and exercise, temperance, and the tonic effects of cold water sharpen the appetite, strengthen the body, set the functions of the skin and the digestion in good order, and react healthfully on the mind. But at the right time, after a duly protracted course of the treatment, certain symptoms and sensations begin, which are often painful both externally and internally; these symptoms are usually (I will not say properly) denominated *crisés*, being as it were the exertions of nature to throw off from the system certain morbid matter. These *crisés*, painful as they are, are expected by the invalids with much impatience, being regarded as sure prognostics that the cold water treatment has been effectual in their complaints, and that they may ultimately be sure of a thorough cure. There is no difficulty in comprehending the theory of these *crisés*, in the following manner, which though of course not positively asserted, appears to me to be the true explanation:—Cold water as a drink dilutes, thins, dissolves, and evacuates: the baths, while they excite the system to reaction, create an irritation on the surface of the body, causing the heat or caloric of the body to fly to the parts subjected to cold water, and thus repair the loss by the sweating; or, since by this Hydropathic process, the surface is exerted and irritated by cold water four or five times a day (supposing we reckon baths, half-baths, douches, &c.), but that the heat and caloric is by these means impelled, without ceasing to the surface, it raises up in the system a centrifugal process, which by degrees attracts the blood and all the humours after the predominating influence of the caloric, and causes them to take the same tendency to the surface. This rush of the liquids of the system to the circumference is so strong that all stagnant matter, all morbid deposits, are of no avail to withstand its influence; and quitting their position, they share in the general perturbation of the system. How, then, is this system to find means of evacuating and exuding so many dangerous and disturbed substances, which, crowding to the surface, collect under the skin, through which they find it impossible to pass? The daily perspirations of Priessnitz alone present the all-excelling assistance which enables Nature by her own efforts to drive from the body those noxious and non-assimilating matters.

"To show how healthful are these perspirations, it is only necessary to run over in our minds the many cases of diseased persons who have been snatched from what seemed (even to medical men) to be inevitable death—and how?—simply by the sudden coming on of a perspiration; a last expiring effort made by the system to give passage through the cutaneous pores to the malignant matter of the disease. Instances of this kind will multiply themselves in the memory of every individual. Speaking of morbid and malignant matter, it may not be amiss to state that at Gräefenberg the bandages after perspiration are often seen impregnated with all kinds of secretions—calcareous, sulphureous, and even metallic—many of them of a disagreeable, fœtid, and sour smell.

"When, however, these perspirations are not strong enough to throw out the required quantity of corrupted matter, or the matter is such that cannot be excreted by perspiration, the skin sooner or later inflames in many places, eruptions are formed, and boils and ulcers show themselves; these burst and throw out corrupt matter in great quantities. Such abscesses are attended with much or little pain, as the case may be, and often heal in one place to burst out in another. In addition to these, owing to the constant excitement, and I may say busy occupation of the system while under the cold-water-treatment, many other symptoms make their appearance, which, as they are attended with fever, assume the appearance to the spectator of danger, and may be considered as critical. These are the symptoms which constitute the true crisis, and it is in his method of treating these, whose violence is a test of the importance and inveteracy of the disease under which the sufferer is labouring, that the tact, the courage, the acuteness, and the master-hand of Priessnitz are to be most seen and admired. It is then, by means of the very cold water that has raised this storm of disease, that he proceeds with calm confidence to allay it, by altering, according to the disease and constitution of the patient, the mode of applying his great remedial applications. Sometimes, in abscesses or fever, he will order the patient to be wrapped in a wet sheet; sometimes he will direct bandages to be put on; sometimes he will send him to a cold bath, or a sitz-bath; sometimes clysters are exhibited; sometimes friction with the hand wetted: now copious draughts of cold water; now a very sparing portion. It is at these times that the character and office of Priessnitz appear most admirable, and it is at these times that a feeling of pain crosses the mind at the thought that Priessnitz alone at present is master of this art of treating the crisis. Let us hope that some enlightened medical men will cast off the prejudices of their schools, and zealous for the good of the whole human race, will study at Grüefenberg to attain the knowledge of this wonderful system, gaining thereby sufficient confidence and skill to treat diseases in their crisis—the most difficult portion, it must be acknowledged by all, of the cold water cure.

"When this crisis is over (and the patient, even at this time, is rarely compelled to keep his bed), then it is that all corrupt matter being driven from the system, the various organs having reassumed the exercise, in a regular manner of their appropriate functions, and the patient being quite out of pain, then it is, I say, that the patient is cured—not of the one disease only for which he came to be treated (let this be most especially noted), but of all and every disease that has been lurking in his system—thoroughly and effectively cured—cleansed of all impurities, and his body once more in a pure and healthy state. Now the doctors can only cure the one complaint under which a sick man suffers, and a hundred others may be latent in his system. Every organ in his body may be deranged in its functions; but the doctors cannot cure them: they know nothing of them; the patient sets down all to his one disease, and therefore complains not of them, and this one disease being cured, a man is often declared well, when his health is neither good nor perfect.

"It is not so with Priessnitz's treatment, for Hydropathy affects the whole system, not one part of the body alone. The water acts generally; it affects all the organs; it rouses up all latent ills; it wakes into action and routs dormant matter; it attacks and remedies all that is morbific and vitiated. Supposing the disease to be incurable, yet, nevertheless, the cold water treatment will strengthen and clear the system, and render more slow its progress. Hence it is that a difficulty arises in saying beforehand how long it will take to effect a cure. Since the length of time required is regulated by the tone of the system, and the special state of each particular organ. This mode of cure by cold water can also be hastened or protracted by the invalid himself, according to the care he takes to support and assist the action of the cold water, by secondary and accessary influences depending on himself, such as pure air, exercise, and food.

"Priessnitz will not take any invalids into his establishment without a prior knowledge of their diseases, some of which he rejects. It is necessary, therefore, to inform him beforehand by letter of the nature of the disease for which you seek relief, lest on arriving at Gräefenberg you be sent back; and this leads me to deliver briefly my sentiments as to the diseases which can be cured by Hydropathy.

"This treatment generally exhibits its salutary effects in a high degree on those who by living too freely, or by the use of spirituous liquors or other excesses, or by a too sedentary life, have weakened their bodies and injured their health; those also who have been in the habit of debilitating their bodies by wearing too many clothes,* and thus become martyrs to rheumatic affections, experience relief in a high degree, and patients of these classes, be their diseases chronic or acute, may make themselves certain of a speedy cure.

" Wonderful cures are also performed by this system in all diseases occasioned by the use of those poisonous drugs, such as mercury, &c., employed in syphilitic complaints. The life led at Gräefenberg, the sweatings, the cold baths, the water drinking, and the fine air, with the exercise taken, all have worked miracles in the way of cure. Syphilitic sufferers who came to Gräefenberg thin, miserable, attenuated, even with a hectic cough, and looking like skeletons, have been seen within a few months, robust, hearty, stout, and lively, and restored to an enjoyment of the pleasures of life.

" Gout, podagra, chiragra, gonagra (feet, hand and knee gouts), sciatica, and all painful complaints proceeding from gout, such as those arising from the settlement of gouty matter in the joints, whence arises what the medical men term anchylosis and contractions, are most successfully treated at Gräefenberg. There is a case of an officer in the Prussian army, who, having become deaf and powerless from gout, was completely cured in the space of nine months.

" By no other method of treatment are abdominal diseases and disorders of the digestive organs so effectually and surely cured. Gastric disorders, as dysentery, cholera, phlegmatic, nervous and intermittent fevers, yield to cold water as a specific, as do piles, hypochondria and hysterics.

" The signal efficacy of this treatment is shown in no cases so much as in abscesses, and ulcers of every kind, especially those having their origin in syphilis or gonorrhœa; caries, too, is even remedied by this treatment. Baron Falkenstein, in his ' Wonders of the Water-cure,' narrates the manner in which he was cured of caries; and a serjeant, whose leg was in such a state of decay as to be condemned to amputation by the doctors, was cured thoroughly by Priessnitz.

" In all inflammatory diseases, internal or external, the cold-water treatment has a most powerful effect. M. Henry, the eminent surgeon, remarks, with respect to internal inflammation, 'If in surgery we find so much advantage from the use of cold water in cases of inflammation, we may ask, why not prefer this remedy which suspends the circulation from any given point, to the practice of treating the disease by internal pathology? Why not give up both general and topical bleeding? It certainly, according to our present notions, seems monstrous to wrap in a wet sheet a patient suffering from inflammation; but this is not enough, this apparent incongruity, to induce us to proscribe a practice of which everyday experience shows the important, beneficial, and speedy effects.'

" In acute diseases of an efflorescent character (as ringworm, erysipelas, &c.), no means prescribed by the pharmacopœia have proved so effectual in assisting the erup-

* M. Priessnitz objects to the wearing flannel and cotton; he maintains, that they weaken the skin, render people delicate, and less able to contend against atmospheric changes. When some one objected to throwing off a flannel waistcoat that he had worn all his life, it being winter, and exceedingly cold, M. Priessnitz said, " wear it, then, over your shirt; but when you are accustomed to cold water you will not miss it. After the bath which you have now taken, run or walk till you provoke perspiration: you need then have no fear of catching cold." Many people are in the habit of wearing flannel waistcoats in the night; this keeps up an unnatural and unnecessary degree of warmth, and increases invisible perspiration, which is unwholesome. Let us look at our gouty and rheumatic subjects, and we shall find that they, perhaps more than other people, have always been accustomed to flannel. Does not this show, that flannel neither protects its wearer from those diseases, nor allays the pain attending them? There are others who are in the habit of clothing the head during night; this is also a practice strongly deprecated at Gräefenberg; it destroys the hair, causes its premature decay, and is highly injurious to persons who are troubled with a flow of blood to the head, headach, colds in the head, &c. There is great sense in the old adage, Keep the head cold, and the feet warm. No people are so much afraid of exposing their heads to the weather as the English. This arises from their habit of sleeping in night caps, and not accustoming themselves to cold ablutions. And a great defect is their being over clothed, so as to exclude the external air. Dr. Abernethy made many experiments as to the effect of the air upon the human body, which have been fully carried out by the late discoveries in hydropathy. It is most probable that the generation of warmth is principally effected by the action of the lungs. The process of perspiration is practised by the skin, if all the pores are open and sound; it therefore results, that to allow the generation of a healthy warmth, a continual activity of the pores of the skin cannot be dispensed with. In proportion as the body is warmly clothed, and the pure air excluded from the skin, the less warmth is produced by the skin itself, and the body becomes chilly, and consequently requires warmer protection. As a healthy naked body generates, by heightened perspiration of the skin, the same warmth as is produced by one which is covered, by means of retaining the perspiration; so every one who is quite well, might, by use, become so hardened, that during the coldest season he might feel, when naked, as comfortable as any one covered with wool. The Scotch Highlander, with his naked legs, does not feel colder, surrounded by mountains of ice, than we who are clothed. We prove this ourselves, by having our faces, bare in the coldest winter.— As the skin performs the double functions,—first, of breathing the air, and drawing nourishment from it; and secondly, of exhaling the phlogisticised air of the diseased matter, and worn-out atoms of the body; it follows, that the true art of curing must be, to endeavour to restore these two functions. Hydropathy causes, by its manifold means of application, the ejection of diseased matter, and the revival of the activity of the skin; and therefore, it makes the principal organ also fit for the second function; viz., that of inhaling the air.—CLARIDGE *on Hydropathy*.

tion as drinking largely of cold water, and the application of cold bandages and the wet sheet, while the skin is hot and dry. In cases where the disease is pronounced incurable this treatment, in its various modifications, will not fail to have a beneficial effect—since if it cannot cure the organs affected, it will, without doubt, strengthen the uninjured portions, so as to enable them the better to stand up against the progress of the cure, and give to Nature, by lapse of time, a further chance, by some of her yet hidden and mysterious processes, which men call accidents, of conquering the disease.

"In conclusion, a word to those who fancy the Hydropathic system can restore youth, and increase or give back the powers of vitality. Neither water nor any other remedy yet discovered can do this—nor does it even cure—it merely sets in motion the powers of the system, and Nature then by her own process effects the cure, by driving out the morbid matter. Nature has thus within her, her own medical powers; water does but arouse, and second the efforts of this power, removing any obstructions which check its progress. If there be nothing to act upon, no remedies can act. Those men who have wasted their vital powers, and decrepit individuals, and individuals whose diseases by inveteracy have already so far triumphed over the energy of the system as to destroy one or more of the organs, must hope in vain to realise in their own persons the brilliant results of this cure.

"To those who have recovered their health at Gräefenberg, I have to recommend great care in not again commencing the intemperate and irrational life they have led before. There are not wanting examples where such an immediate renewal of an irregular life, after a most successful cure, has occasioned a sudden death. Nature will not be trifled with. On going from Gräefenberg, wisdom and prudence must be observed; a fixed and regulated restraint must be exercised in diet, and the Gräefenberg treatment observed as far, at least, as regards the drinking and frequent washing in cold water.

"As for myself, I left Gräefenberg after a sojourn of sixteen days, restored to health, a time which, though brief, will remain ever deeply engraven in my memory. Though perfectly cured, I still, nevertheless, keep up the practice of the outward and inward application of cold water; and although by no means particular, or bound to any minute regulation of diet, I endeavour to preserve moderation in the pleasures and enjoyments of life. If I feel ill, I fast strictly and drink cold water continually. This method of living keeps me in perfect health, makes me feel brisk, strong and gay, and indeed I must say that I am quite as much of a youth as any man can boast of being at the age of fifty-three."

Such is the account given of the cold-water treatment by an intelligent eye-witness; and supposing that our readers have now obtained some partial insight into the theory, principle, and practice of hydropathy, we shall proceed to place it more fully within their comprehension.

THE SYSTEM AND THEORY OF THE COLD WATER CURE.

The system of Hydropathy, or Cold Water Treatment, and its theory, as deduced by Priessnitz from observation and experience, we find to be as follows:—

I. Health is the true and natural condition of the body.

II. A diseased condition of the body may proceed from external injury, such as burns, cuts, bruises, &c.; but these, in a healthy state of the body, will heal of themselves by simple applications, except where requiring the aid of the surgeon, or rather bone-setter.

III. Disease is also produced by foreign matters absorbed or introduced into the system.

IV. These matters, alien to the system and prejudicial to its health, are—
1. Substances formed in a natural manner, by the usual secretions and processes of the animal functions, but which have not been carried off or evaporated at the due time.
2. Substances which have no assimilation* with the human body, and which, by fortuitous circumstances, have found their way into the stomach, or through the skin, or upon it.
3. A bad state of the elements, water and air, producing epidemics.
4. Ulcerations and contagious disease, as syphilis, &c.

* There is something so curious, so instructive, and so ingenious in Mr. Claridge's observations on this portion of the subject that we cannot but insert them:—
"ASSIMILATION.—To attain the preservation of life, it is required not only that its consumption should be reduced, but that its restoration should be rendered more easy. For this purpose two things are most essentially necessary,—the perfect assimilation of that which may be of benefit, and the separation of that which may be injurious; for life depends, as will be seen by the following definition, upon the identification, the assimilation, and the animalisation of external matter, in its passage from the chemical to the organic world by the vital power. The power of assimilating other substances into itself is the fundamental principle of nature; this impulse and power is not only prevalent in all organic matter, but also in elemental bodies, that is to say, water, earth, and fire. The globe in the beginning was a rigid rock, upon which the air and the water effected their power of assimilation. Assimilation is only possible by dissolving; for the purpose of assimilating, air and water dissolved the earth's crust, by the agency of which powers that surface originated, which produces and nourishes all organic bodies; as these exist in the same world in which the elements continually exercise their power of dissolving and assimilating. It follows that from the beginning there must have been developed in all organic

V. Disease assumes an acute form when the system makes an effort to drive out the corrupt or non-assimilating matter.

VI. Fever is not disease, but is produced by it, when the system has exerted itself beyond its power in expelling the diseased matter.

VII. An acute disease can only be extirpated by dissolving the diseased matter by the agency of water—a means which never fails to effect that object in such a manner as even to be perceptible to the senses.

VIII. Physic and bleeding render permanent or chronic all acute diseases. Medical treatment seldom finally ejects the diseased matter from the system, though a partial cure may apparently be effected. Hence physicians can never arrive accurately by their system at the true and latent first causes of any disease.

IX. A continuance in a course of drugs must in the end, either sooner or later, paralyse the powers of the system, and make the body yield to their effects.* Hence, whoever suffers from chronic disease can never die a natural death; unless, before it be too late, he resorts to hydropathy for a final cure, which changes the chronic disease, by disturbing the corrupt and diseased matter, and drives it out of the body by acute eruptions, thus changing the chronic to an acute disease, which it cures in the same manner as an acute disease is cured at first, viz., by the cold-water treatment.

X. According to the intentions and institutions of nature, as revealed by the organisation of man, he should, if he lived according to her laws, enjoy a life without pain, and die a natural death, unaccompanied by suffering or pain. Yet what do we see

---

elements the same power as a protection to themselves. Air dissolves water into vapours, in order to assimilate gases from it. Water again extracts from air the oxygen gas. Fire absorbs the oxygen of air, it dissolves water into its two component parts, hydrogen and oxygen, and by converting the former to a flame, it transforms water to fire; air absorbs many gases which fire releases from combustibles; air draws gases from the soil, the soil absorbs the oxygen of the air. In this way the elements are in a constant conflict, each endeavouring to dissolve the other, and to assimilate its matters with itself. Organic bodies draw the oxygen from the air by the process of respiration, which is also the property of plants; these draw all assimilatory matter which the earth offers by their roots, and the same process is performed by animals feeding on plants or herbs; whereas, on the contrary, fire dissolves and assimilates to itself all organic matter. This same process is carried out by water and air, with all organic beings, but as long as these are living they only get their evaporation, and after death their entirety. The earth exercises this power but conditionally and partially, viz., upon all animals that exist in it, and on all roots of plants; upon mankind the earth only exercises its power of assimilation after death. The proofs of this conflict of assimilation amongst organic matter itself are very clear, one animal eats the other as well as plants; that is to say, it absorbs by the agency of the stomach so much of their substance as may be assimilated; plants again convert many parts of dead bodies and other plants (the manure) into their own substance. Besides this power of assimilation, there exists in every being, element and organisation, the necessity of being exposed to foreign assimilation. This is the fundamental principle of the true doctrine of healing. In support of this theory we find that water, if withdrawn from the power of dissolution by the fresh air, stinks and putrefies; air loses its quantity of oxygen, and becomes mephitic, if it does not find water or plants with which it can enter into the conflict of dissolution and assimilation."—*Claridge's Hydropathy*, p. 127.

* By what delusions were mankind, in the first instance, persuaded to submit to the use of poisonous drugs? In the middle ages, the use of water as a drink, and a cure for disease, fell into total disuse, when, in the time of the Crusade, the Arab doctors introduced the use of Oriental drugs, to which they attributed miraculous virtues; and during the period of astrology and alchymy, and when such assiduous researches were made for the philosophers' stone, almost every nation boasted of having found some panacea, some elixir vitæ; sometimes it was an oil or a herb, at others, a powder or mineral, until, in process of time, these accumulated in such numbers, that the administration of them formed a science. But, we would inquire, are the effects of these compounds such as to lead us to conclude, that they were recommended by nature? Have mankind become healthier since their introduction? No, quite the contrary. Are those nations who have done most homage to this science, the strongest and soundest? No; for they are, beyond contradiction, physically, if not morally, the most miserable of all. Again, we would ask, are those individuals amongst them who do most to aid the apothecaries healthier than the others? or, are those who constantly consult doctors free from pain? We have the same answer, No; their lives are worse than death. But if we did not know to the contrary, we should certainly conclude that doctors are healthy. This may fairly be expected from future water doctors, otherwise, like the rest, they would manifest their incompetency in their own persons. No one seems to reflect that at least a doctor ought to be able to cure himself. We are so accustomed to illness and wretchedness that we consider it a necessary part of this life, and are the less disposed to complain, since the masters of physic suffer very seriously from its effects themselves. Some writers suppose mankind have arrived at an age of decrepitude; but in this they err, from its not occurring to them that the lamentable state of public health arises from art and not nature. If you wish to be convinced of this, go to the forests of savages. There you will see that the present man of nature is as young and strong as the first who was created; the generation cannot grow old, except by art, poison, or vice. Prescribe simple spring water, and it is rejected with scorn; but let any quack recommend his drugs, however poisonous, and they are swallowed and paid for on the instant. One would suppose that it must have been the Enemy of all Good only, that could have first persuaded mankind that poison could produce health. The evils that arise from pernicious drugs, which have swept away millions, and which will destroy the whole species if no reform take place, originate in misunderstanding the first or acute disease, which is but an attempt of nature to heal. Men took the symptoms of fever for the disease itself, and being relieved by bleeding, blistering, and drugs, they praised the unlucky discovery. From this cause a host of deadly diseases took their origin, such as destructions and suppurations of the inner organs, dropsy, &c., diseases which were hardly known in times of yore, and which would never have reared their heads but for the poisonous effects of drugs and the general distaste for water, the only element prescribed by nature. However, as the lamentable consequences do not appear until, perhaps, years after the suppression of the acute conflict have elapsed, no one thinks of accusing drugs as the cause.—*Claridge on Hydropathy*.

B

daily?—men dying not naturally; not from gradual decay of strength and wasting of the body and its powers; but from the poison of drugs ignorantly administered as medicines; liquors that make drunken and inflame; food adulterated with non-assimilating matter; want of water, at the very contact of which men seem to tremble like patients with the hydrophobia; corrupted air from man's own sloth, in not frequently renewing it by some healthful change of place, and want of exercise. Natural causes of ill-health are but three. First, that the naturally assimilating elements may be corrupted, as air or water, and thus are deteriorated the two principal requisites of health, and epidemics ensue. To these men and animals are alike exposed. Contagious diseases also are another natural source of ill-health; but, except from these, no man who lives upon the natural water regime need ever dread the attacks of illness. With the exception of accidental wounds, contagion and epidemy, as before specified, and even from these may he be cured speedily and effectually in retaining his health afterwards, the same as before, which can be said of no system of medical treatment by drugs.

XI. What wise man, then, would think of curing one disease with drugs which inevitably bring on another: for how can that physic be brought to act upon the diseased matter, dispersed as it is, and hidden in the deep and secret recesses of the system? and could this even be effected, how can the two matters, the drugs and the disease, unite, coalesce, and dissolve each other into *nothing*? A residuum must be left-behind as every chemist knows; and therein lies the evil—to the old disease a new morbific stimulant is added, weak or strong, according to the nature and qualities of the drugs administered.

XII. No cure, either of men, animals or plants, can be effectual without the aid of air and water, the grand dissolving elements.

XIII. The cold water treatment is the one which nature has placed in the power of all her creatures; and without water taken inwardly and applied outwardly, there can be no health. Nature has no secrets in giving man life, she has implanted within him the knowledge of and the capacity for what is to support and render pleasant that life. Nature has no mysteries: her blue heavens, her green fields, and her running-stream, which give pleasure to the senses, will also, if they be properly used, give health and recreation to the body.

Such, in a few words, is the system, and such the theory of M. Priessnitz. We shall now proceed with this as our theme to enlarge upon, and by due examples and illustrations to bring it more clearly to the understanding and comprehension of those of our readers, who may wish to learn sufficient of this most admirable system to practise it as far as possible in their own families.

All diseases have their origin in a derangement of the organs which operate in keeping up life and health. To form an estimate of diseases by their names and the various phases in which they show themselves, we should find almost numberless. By deducing them to the causes from which they spring, they will be greatly lessened in number. Multiplicity of form does not imply multiplicity of causes. It is the result of a diversity of organs, each of which has its separate functions to perform. Water, air, climate, repose, exercise, wakefulness, food, drink, sleep, and the passions, are the elements of moral and physical life. The preservation of these in exact equilibrium preserves health; their inequality therein is the source of disease. Pure air and water, and the salubrity of the place or climate he inhabits, are not always at man's command; but exercise or repose, vigilance or sleep, are at his own choice; so are his food and drink, and reason is at hand to control his passions. Gluttony is set down by religion as one of the seven capital sins. Medicine, not to be behind, sets it down as the occasion of many diseases, and the aggravation of those it does not occasion. "I leave behind me," said a celebrated physician on his deathbed, "two great physicians, diet and water." Who has not cured a slight illness, and prevented a serious one in its origin, by diet and cold water? In either chronic or acute diseases, the medical man sets to work to cleanse the primary ducts by vomitings, sweating, and purgings: he introduces in the second, remedies to aid nature's work, whose servant only he knows himself to be. *Priessnitz does the very same with water, Water is the greatest dissolvent in nature.* If the primary ducts be obstructed, water dilutes, attenuates, divides, and scatters the impurities contained in them; and these are afterwards ejected by the stomach and intestines. He uses cold water, because that temperature is tonic and fortifying, and gives to nature an additional energy in expelling the diseased matter. If the disease be settled in the blood, and the morbific matter deposited in the different organs of the animal economy, what better than water can dilute the thickened and blunt the acute; revivify what languishes, extinguish what burns, and open again all the passages by which injurious humours can escape? A sudorific process, unknown until Priessnitz's time, produces perspiration, without wearying the organic system. It is supported by copious draughts of cold water, which quench the thirst, moisten and refresh the blood, replace the lost juices, and maintain the tone of the muscles. The cold bath into which the body, in a state of perspiration, is plunged, is exempt from any possibility of producing agitation of respiration or circulation, giving back to the skin the tone and energy which it had lost by perspiration. The exercise following this restores to the body the lost heat. There is not one single instance of any person catching cold, produced by these sudden transitions from heat to cold;— a phenomenon easily explained, from the general calm and equilibrium of the system.

The douche bath is intended to disturb the acrid juices identified with the organs, and cause them to come out on the skin, which is stimulated by its blows. Local baths have the same object: hip-baths and foot-baths have the property of drawing humours away from the head and chest. Heating, or wet linen bandages, are sometimes covered with dry linen, sometimes not. The former are continually applied to weak parts, or those labouring under obstruction. The purpose of all these processes together is to convey the morbid humours to the skin, whence they exude in eruptions, boils, and abscesses. These eruptions, constituting the crisis of the complaint, are the certain sign of a perfect cure. After the unwholesome juices are driven out and replaced by wholesome ones, then follow the restoration of the digestive powers, the freeing of all the organs by the dissolving of all obstructions, the vital and animal functions are re-established in their former harmony; nothing then remains but health, a treasure which can only be preserved by continuing the system to which is owing its acquirement. The mission of all medicine is to ease pain, calm irritation, and allay the burning heat, which are concomitant with inflammation and fever; to moisten, dilute, and attenuate all that is dry, thick, and hardened; to soften down acrimony, to remove obstructions; to dissipate congestions; to keep open all the excretory passages; to attract therein all hurtful humours, and effect their discharge; lastly, to maintain the invalid's strength as required by nature, which itself labours in this great work, the accomplishment of which it is the duty of medicine to assist and not impede. If it be objected that one remedy cannot fulfil so many various objects, we reply, that it is multiplied by those acquainted with its use; that the numerous methods in which it is employed answer to the numerous remedies which art would produce. For foot-baths, half-baths, partial and entire baths, the douche and injections, although all consisting of cold water, are so many distinct remedies, each having its particular properties answering to the different kinds of assistance which nature may require. Nor can it be said with propriety that this curative process has but one remedy, whilst the eminently powerful and beneficial sudorific process is put in requisition; nor should exercise, the restraint of the appetite to wholesome and simple food, and the silence of passions, be looked upon as of no remedial importance. The absence of excitement from the pleasures of society, is also another means, which like the other methods of this process as it can be everywhere proved, is within the reach of all. Such then being the case, medical science comes down at the command of common sense and experience from the height to which she has so long been raised, and we must drown all the learning of the doctors in that element with which the Author of nature has thought fit to cover three parts of the globe. We must shut up that immense store-house of medicaments which chemical and botanical ingenuity have drawn from the three kingdoms of nature and the four quarters of the world, and put on one side as worthless the fruit of so many labours; the heir-loom of so many ages; the whole materiel in short, on which the temple of Esculapius has been raised. And this, for what? to give to suffering mankind but one remedy for all their numerous ills, to confine them to one panacea, one grand universal remedy—cold water! Can we then wonder at the outcry of opposition which has been raised against our system, an outcry of violent passion and selfish interests; an outcry, which nothing but the experience of the last fifteen years in Germany, and the favourable report of a high commission sent down (with all the prejudices of art against a new system) have alone been able to subdue.

The learned must lay aside their science, the practitioner give up his connexion, the apothecary throw his drugs to his dogs, for Nature has at last disclosed to a mountain peasant, and through him to the world, her great secret, which sages, philosophers, physicians, and kings so long sought for in their alchymical studies. Thanks to Priessnitz, who never heard of Galen or Hippocrates, we now know no other remedy than water, air, exercise, and diet. Our theory is now, for the first time, a written one. We require to feel no pulses, to examine no tongues; neither diagnostics nor prognostics are necessary. Medical aliments we throw on one side—food and drink alone occupy our attention, which we look upon, in conjunction with the air, as the materials of the human body, perpetually entering into its substance, composing and recomposing it. When wholesome, and used proportionately with our wants, they are natural supports and creators of our health; when unwholesome, when taken without moderation, what are they but the engenders of disease? Air is to the lungs what food is to the stomach. Respiration is not a voluntary function: a man must breathe whether he will or not; or he must die. He eats, then, and he breathes; but Nature, who has given him the power of moving, demands that he should do more—he should take exercise, without which digestion languishes, the blood gets sluggish in its flow, the mind and the body become torpid, and life is merely vegetation. The citizen and the countryman have been not inaptly likened—the one to a plant placed in a hot-house, of a dwindled and unhealthy growth; the other to the same plant shooting up in the open ground, under the influence of a life-inspiring sun-lit air. It has been said by naturalists, that the motion of the air is necessary to the health of plants; the wind, thus, is the exercise of vegetable life. Let man, then, follow their example; but more fortunate than they, he has not to wait for rain to quench his thirst: for him the liquid element flows in almost every plain. How surprising is the little use he makes of it, both externally and internally! Behold him, for ambition and for gain, reduce and expand it to steam, and work every day new miracles with it. See, does he spare it to his kitchen-garden and his flower-beds? He knows that water is their nourishment, and preserves the fresh lustre and painted beauty of his flowers. In fact, he uses this element in every way but the proper one.

By what evil genius, then, are his eyes blinded to its great hygeian virtues? Let us own, with Vincent Priessnitz, that it is because he hates what is simple, and thirsts after what is difficult and complexed, a victim to his pride and his sensuality. Ere arts were invented, water was man's only beverage. Ancient history is full of the reputation of those prophylactic institutions which the generosity and hospitality of ancient manners threw open to all. There were then public baths without tax or price, and the people thronged to them in crowds. To what shall we ascribe that great strength which made the Romans fit conquerors of the world, but to the general use of baths? *Nec degere nec natare didicit* was then, indeed, a reproach, and proves the frequency of the bath. How can we without wonder behold their armour, which no warrior of our day could support on his valiant shoulders? How soon did opulence, torn from the spoils of vanquished cities, alter the primal simplicity of nature! No longer did simple pleasures content the senses. The appetite was doubled by the invention of a refined cookery, and stimulated by sauces and sharpened by seasonings, which nature never designed for human stomachs. Hence the digestive organs, unused to new sensations, and laden overmuch by juices forced into existence in too great richness and quantity, became deranged, the functions grew discordant, and diseases sprang up which were hitherto unheard of and unknown. Motion became tiresome, its powers weakened by this derangement and excitement; and hence came reluctance first, and then inability to take the necessary exercise. The economy of the system lost its equilibrium. It was now that warm-baths, as better suited to the over-excitement of the sensitive system, took the place of cold-baths, muscular strength was lost, weakness and disease took the place of strength, and health fled the civilised world to more barbaric regions where temperance is honoured and observed. What, then, remains but as far as possible to revert back to a natural system, and at once adopt and follow out the practice of the cold water cure?

PRACTICE OF THE COLD WATER CURE.

The Hydropathical method of treating diseases is comprised in a peculiar regimen; in the use of great quantities of cold water as a drink; in arousing the system; in copious and frequent perspirations; in the use of entire and local cold-baths, cold ablutions, and injections; of frictions, douches, and cold wet fomentations or heating bandages. The value of regimen in the curing of all diseases is too well known to render it incumbent on us to enter into details on that subject. We therefore shall confine ourselves to the observation, that if a particular diet be necessary in the treatment of acute diseases, it is not less so in the treatment of chronic complaints; since it is only in the debilitating habits of a sedentary life, in the excess of mental occupation, in richness of food, in the too frequent use of fermented liquors, in the corrupt air of towns, and the harassings of domestic life, that the great majority of chronic diseases have their origin. When such persons seek to regain their health, they must give up all these causes, at any rate so long as they place themselves under the cold water treatment.

The drinking of cold water, in large quantities, acts especially upon the stomach and all the digestive organs. Its particular temperature causes contractions of greater power, refreshes the stomach and intestines by dissolving all obstructions, and gives them tone without irritation. All who give its due value to digestion in the curing of chronic diseases, will at once estimate at its true price the service which cold water may render. This neutral fluid being easily absorbed, renders the blood more fluid; and having, through the circulation, obtained an entrance into the interior of the organs, it there dissolves all excretory matter—water, whenever it passes off, either as urine or by perspiration, being strongly impregnated with impure or excretory matter.

Cold water, as a beverage, makes its way more freely into the intestines than any other remedy. By its property of dilutation, it aids all evacuations without forcing them, and the system has the power of choosing its own way and time.

SWEATING.—This method of treatment is to invest the body in blankets, and so hinder the escape of the caloric of the human frame. These perspirations do not differ from the ordinary ones, but the morbid matter when dissolved, exudes through the skin: sometimes it is coloured green or yellow, and throws off unpleasant odours: it is even sometimes fetid. This is in itself a curious phenomenon for pathological inquirers to notice the different odours arising from perspiration, after certain medicines, such as mercury and sulphur, have been taken, even though several years have elapsed. Critical sweats have, in patients who have taken mercury, the same fetid smell which occurs on mercurial salivation; and those who have used sulphur exhale a smell of that substance. Those perspirations are called critical when the invalid is visibly relieved.

The concentration of organic heat excites the blood and lymph, and makes them circulate more rapidly in the capillary vessels. The casting out of the excretory substances dissolved by the cold water, taken as a drink, is made more copious from the skin, assisted as it is by a quickened circulation; and as a corrective of that weakness of the body which results from the open state of the capillary vessels; creating, as we see in the colliquative sweats, a free exit not only for the morbid and diseased parts, but also to the nourishing matter, and those necessary for the system, ablutions and cold baths are made use of. These must be taken gradually, descending from 72 to 45 degrees. By their temperature they cause a contraction in the capillary vessels, prevent the skin becoming too sensitive to atmospheric changes (as is the case from the prolonged use of warm baths); they cleanse the epidermis from the perspiration, and, by their action, stimulate in a high degree a reaction of the system. It is well known, that after the application of one of these agents people become warm, even in a low degree of temperature.

We must now disperse the fears which a great number of persons entertain (and which we only ourselves got the better of after seeing for some months the wonderful effects of the cure at Gräefenberg on more than six thousand patients of all ages, sexes, and constitutions) through their drinking or bathing in cold water when heated, or even when the body is covered with perspiration. For though, if we give faith to medical men, the experience of centuries seems to prove that thousands of persons have been subjected to inflammation of the lungs, heart, head, liver, and to apoplexy, after drinking cold water when heated, or in a state of perspiration; yet, nevertheless, on the contrary, every day at Gräefenberg hundreds of persons, bathed with perspiration, are seen drinking plentifully of cold water, and while in that state plunging into a cold bath, without, out of ten thousand persons who have visited Gräefenberg since the discovery of Hydropathy, a single instance of injury arising from such treatment.

And how much more assured may we be of the beneficial effects of this treatment when a Government so cautious as the Austrian Government, jealous almost to a fault of the health of their subjects, and with a medical police severe to an extreme, gives every encouragement to this treatment, in the full conviction and persuasion that it is not only without danger, but fraught with the greatest blessings to the health of the community?

To comprehend these apparently contradictory facts, let us inquire into the manner in which these perspirations, so decidedly different in their effects, are produced. When perspiration is brought on by medicines or exertion, such as dancing or other fatiguing movements, the skin not only perspires, but the action of the respiratory organs and the circulation are strongly accelerated; and the radical viscera of life, the brain, heart, and lungs, are all in a state of excitement; such is not the case in sweats brought on through the treatment at Gräefenberg, which concentrates the heat in the body by blankets, and excites the action of the skin, without any movement on the part of the patient. The skin alone is here irritated, as is proved by its redness and its heat, whilst the internal organs are refreshed by cold water, given at that time with the view of keeping up the perspiration.

The use of the douche-bath at first creates violent excitement, by causing throughout the whole body a strong reaction, owing in part to the mechanical action of water falling from 10 to 18 feet, and in part by its coldness; these produce a redness of the skin, and give heat, activity, and strength to the body, as well as an additional power of action to the digestive functions. The douches are prescribed when it is wished to create a strong reaction, to fortify the skin, to dissipate the accumulation of morbid and inert deposits by exciting their absorption, as in cases of swelling of the glands and joints; they are also efficacious in throwing out again upon the surface ringworms, which had been thrown into the system; they occasion also a critical hemorrhage and discharge of hemorrhoids, and rouse to activity the venous and capillary circulation in the abdominal obstructions. From these details, we can understand that the douche is injurious in those cases where the reaction of the blood and nerves requires to be diminished or calmed. The primary effect of the sitz and foot baths is a feeling of cold in the parts submitted to the action of water, and a congestion to the upper regions of the body. This we can prevent by the application of a cold wet cloth to the head during the first ten minutes. By withdrawing from the body all its superfluous heat, the water soon loses its low temperature and becomes warm. At first the parts wetted are alone refreshed, but very soon the whole mass of blood, which by the rapidity of its circulation, passes and repasses to and from the cold parts, gives warmth to them, and so, by gradual circulation, the upper part of the body also becomes refreshed.

When the patient has been some time in a sitz bath the pulse slackens, and the blood congested to the head descends, by reaction, to the lower portion of his body; thus headachs, inflamed eyes, toothachs, and sore throats, experience relief. This method is milder and more certain than the immediate application of cold water to the head, since the reaction which follows that application, if it be not continued, increases, by its secondary action, the congestion which it had calmed by its first.

The action of cold sitz and foot-baths lessens congestions of blood to the upper regions of the body, by the reaction of the system which follows from them, and accelerates the capillary circulation of the parts immersed. Hence their advantage in hemorrhoids, diarrhœa, &c. But when intestine inflammations are to be remedied, or dysentery, or chronic diarrhœa, sitz-baths, with the chill off, 64° Fah., are employed at first. In these the patient remains for hours, the water being changed every half hour, each time a little colder, until it becomes very cold. During the whole time copious draughts of cold water must be taken in small quantities at a time until shivering comes on, and the whole body soon after becomes thoroughly refreshed.

As sitz-baths are more generally used, and may be considered milder than entire baths or ablutions, which can only be employed for a few minutes, every invalid who, wishes to follow the practice adopted at Gräefenberg, should use them once or twice a day. Friction with the hand stimulates the circulation of the blood in the abdomen.

As a neutral fluid, water permeates through the body, as in a filter; and is of the same importance to the human system as to all nature, where it operates to dissolve and facilitate compositions and decompositions, after the maxim of physicians, "*corpora non agunt nisi soluta,*" bodies will not act unless in a state of solution; and when we take into consideration that all matter in the system derives its principle from the blood, which becomes fluid after being used by the organs of life, before it is emitted from the body, it must be acknowledged that water, which facilitates this fluidity, must assist circulation in the more delicate vessels of the body, and by that means effectually aids in the reparation and reproduction, and as it were recreation of it as the material parts composing our system.

As regards its temperature, the effects of water are different under different circumstances, dependent upon a long or short time of application; that is to say, whether we use it for its first or secondary action; whether we are to be warmed by the caloric of the body withdrawn from it into the water or to be kept cold by frequent renewal of the water. Again, its action differs when applied to a part afflicted, from its operation on a part distant from the locality of the disease. The primary effect of water is sudden, and then gives place to a secondary effect, which is reaction; and those who wash themselves with cold water, or have rubbed themselves with snow, can testify to this as a fact of daily occurrence.

Is, then, the cold water treatment at Gräefenberg applicable to all descriptions of disease? We answer, that its application must be of advantage in the large number of acute and chronic diseases. Cases there are, however, wherein, some essential organ having become defective, art can do no more than prolong existence and alleviate suffering. Among such exceptions are consumption, organic diseases of the heart, of the lungs, of the large vessels, dropsy, &c. Nevertheless, even all these cases, and others confessed on all sides to be incurable, by the moderate use of some of the cold water applications, will, if judiciously employed, ensure relief and palliation of pain.

But will cold water treatment ensure a radical cure? What are we to understand by the word radical? If by it be meant the final rooting out from the system that which has caused disease, and the relief of the patient from pain, then, indeed, the cure by the cold water method is *radical!* But if to be radical, a cure is sought which is to prevent a return of the disease, in cases of parties exposing themselves to the same influences as originally caused the disease, then most certainly neither this nor any other method of treatment will have such an effect.

As to danger from the cold water treatment of Gräefenberg, we do not believe that there can be any active mode of treatment more innocent, with reference to its present or future effects, provided only it be applied with judgment; but if it be injudiciously used, it may not improbably be attended with dangerous consequences.

People ignorant of Hydropathy fancy that the drinking plentifully of cold water has a tendency to bring on dropsy. We will speedily convince them of their error in this respect. It is not water which causes dropsy, but a watery albuminous fluid, generally coagulated by heat and acids. This fluid, in dropsical patients, fills up the cellulary tissue and the different cavities of the body, and is produced by a morbid secretion of the watery membranes which line the interior of the cavities. This secretion is caused by the irritation of the membranes, and results from the abuse of fermented liquors. Cold water, in whatever quantities it may be drank, could not possibly produce this secretion. Others say, that this novel mode of cure will shrivel the skin, make wrinkles, and cause people to look much older than they really are: this is not less unfounded. True, indeed, it is, that warm baths and hot climates weaken and relax the contractibility of the skin, and certainly bring on wrinkles prematurely. On the other hand, also, intense and continual cold, as in northern regions, prevents the full development of the body, and contracts the surface, producing a like result; but the action of cold-baths is momentary, and produces quite different results, giving tone and contractibility to the skin. Does not the reaction produced by cold, in attracting the blood, by capillary action to the surface, maintain, by its more active circulation, the nourishment and healthy colour of the skin, and facilitate the excretory process, and prevent the heating of that organ? No; so far from making wrinkles, cold water is the most certain method to prevent them. Experience tells us, that to the use of cold baths and cold water, as a drink, thousands of persons owe the preservation of their freshness of skin and colour to a very advanced age. This fact completely justifies the opinion expressed by numerous celebrated physicians, that cold water is the best of all cosmetics.

It is now necessary that we give such an account of the practice of M. Priessnitz and his various methods of applying this only element of his pharmacopœia, cold water, as may enable those of our readers who cannot visit his establishment at Gräefenberg, to apply their knowledge obtained from this little book, to useful purposes in their own home: and first it may be necessary to premise that

THE WATER

at Gräefenberg has no advantage over that which is to be met with everywhere. It is, however, particularly cold and fresh. For the purposes of the cold-water cure, water must be what is called "soft:" i. e., it must have the quality of dissolving, and therefore must be cold and without any mineral properties. To prove its fitness, linen cloth washed in it must become white, and vegetables dressed in it must be tender. Trout living in water is not a proof of its softness, but frogs are. Hard water makes the skin rough; soft water, on the contrary, renders it smooth.

SWEATING AND THE BATH.

ADVANTAGES OF SWEATING.—This part of the hydropathic process is, to say the best of it, unpleasant; but practice soon removes much of its unpleasantness. The position in which the patient is kept, and the irritation resulting, are at first disagreeable; but when the perspiration begins, a pleasant relief is felt, which the sun freely admitted at the windows tends greatly to increase. Perspiration is at once the most prominent, as it is the most frequent, of the evacuations which tend to the relief of disease; and the main advantage of the new process introduced by Vincent Priessnitz is, that it does not stimulate the blood like other sudorific processes. Unlike vapour baths, which excite the organs of perspiration extremely, the hydropathic process leaves them calm and tranquil; the cold water refreshes the blood and prevents congestion to the head or chest, while the fresh air fails not to calm any slight irritation. Such being the advantage of this sweating process, it is plain to the humblest capacity that such is its efficacy as to enable it to be employed for days and months without weakening the system. This at once shows how it is possible to cure, by sweating, diseases of the most inveterate nature. Those who have witnessed its application at Gräefenberg, can bear testimony to the innumerable cures it has effected, from which the public can judge of its great and real importance. We see it more especially in the division, dissolving, and alternation of the humours which its stimulating properties draw to the skin; while the cold bath following after, strengthens the tone and invigorates the energies of the system and the circulation of the blood, and drives out all the stagnant humours. This process is the grand characteristic of M. Priessnitz's method of treatment; and to this process we submit all disorders having their origin in the vitiated juices.

THE METHOD OF THE SWEATING PROCESS.—The patient is wrapped naked in a large thick blanket, the arms close to the body, the legs stretched out; the blanket is then rolled round the body as tight as it can be, and turned under at the feet; on this is placed a small feather-bed, such as are used in Germany instead of blankets on the bed, in default of which an extra pair of blankets will answer the same purpose; over these a sheet and counterpane are spread, and the patient lies covered up looking like a mummy in its multiplied coverings. The head may be covered also (if there be no tendency of blood to the head) in cases where it appears difficult to bring on perspiration. The close confinement, the length of time, and the irritating influence of the blanket on the skin, make this in general not a very pleasant operation to endure, although the irritation goes off when perspiration comes on; this, however, seldom happens under three-quarters of an hour, or sometimes even two hours. In this state (when the perspiration is on) the patient must remain from half an hour to two hours, according to the nature of the complaint. When the patient is first *packed up*, a urinal is deposited between his legs, and wet cloths are wrapped round any diseased part. Those who are slow to perspire, are advised to keep their legs in as much motion as possible, and rub their body with their hands, moving as much as their compressed condition will allow. Exertion, however, is not desirable, and it is to be rather avoided than encouraged. Perspiration is slower to come on in summer than in winter. As soon as it has begun, all the windows in the room must be opened, and a glass of cold water given to the patient every half hour, not only to refresh him, but also to encourage the sweating, which it does greatly. If headach be felt during the process, a damp cloth may be wrapped round the head, and it will relieve it without fail. The length of time which the sweating is to endure, is a matter in which M. Priessnitz exhibits great skill and powers of discriminating between cases; some are made to sweat every day, some on alternate days, and others once only in three days. Nor let any one suppose that this constant sweating tends to make the patients lean, thin, and weak; on the contrary, men who sweated every day were observed to have lost neither weight nor strength, and indeed, in the latter, they had improved wonderfully, as well as in their personal appearance. In general, it may be known when the sweating has continued sufficiently long, by the breaking out of the perspiration on the patient's face. The attendant is now summoned, and all the bed-clothes are taken off, except the blanket, in this the invalid is to go the bath. He is now supplied with a pair of straw slippers, and the face, legs, and all parts likely to be exposed to the action of the air, are wiped down by the attendant with a wet cloth. The blanket is drawn round the body, and over the head, and in this manner the patient marches to the bath, which, of course, is always near, either in the next room, or the one underneath. After washing the top of the head, face, neck, and chest, he then goes into the bath, and remains there from ten to eight minutes, as he may be advised. In this the theory of M. Priessnitz is diametrically opposed to that of those who enjoin that a body heated and in perspiration should be carefully guarded from exposure to cold; and yet, strange to say, both the doctors and M. Priessnitz's are in the right. The former in shunning cold when the body is heated by motion, or excited by sudorifics, for, in such a case, death would surely follow such exposure; but by the hydropathic system, neither are the organs of circulation or perspiration stimulated, by motion or by drugs, quite on the contrary, they are calm and undisturbed. Moreover, the skin comes in contact not with mere dry cold air, but it is by the stimulating effect of cold water on the surface of the body, in a state of perspiration. The irritation ensuing re-acts, and produces a heat, which a dry cold from the air does not, and hence a fine redness of the skin should be seen in all hydropathic patients on coming out of the bath. This redness should also be observable after the douche, and it is to the doctor and the patient a sure diagnostic; to the one it shows that the patient has sufficient strength to fight against the disease, in the other it inspires a well-grounded hope of restoration to perfect health. It proves an activity in the vessels of the skin, and by the growth and strength of this activity is judged the proximity or distance of the final cure. Perspirations at night, which tend to weaken the system, are to be avoided. This can be done by letting the bed-clothes be light, and washing the body at night with cold water. If the functions of the skin appear to be deranged, it may be necessary to wrap the patient in a wet sheet, before covering him up for sweating—this gives tone to the skin. The sweating process must, however, be used with great care—and here we must beg our readers' strict attention to the rules laid down in the method of curing diseases, which follows immediately this branch of our subject. At Gräefenberg not one half of the patients are allowed to be sweated; and, in these cases, M. Priessnitz uses the greatest discrimination.

ABLUTIONS.—When the patient is extremely weak, he is washed all over, in place of the bath or douche; and in cases of feverish irritability water is poured on the head, and thus the whole body is wetted. It is then rubbed with the hand, first all over, and then on the parts affected. If the patient be too weak to allow of this rubbing, a wet sheet is thrown over him, on which the friction is applied. This is of great advantage in weak cases and young children. The ablutions are an essential, agreeable, and valuable portion of the cold water system; and those who wish to be their own cold water doctors, cannot do better than pay great attention to them. The best time for them is on rising in the morning, and at night before bed. In minor complaints, and even in those more serious, at their first commencement—in gout in the early stages, or nervous irritation, these ablutions will often of themselves, if plenty of cold water is also drunk, be enough to restore health. After the morning ablutions, to be taken instantly on getting out of bed, before the body is chilled, the patient must not fail to go out for exercise. To use the wet sheet as an ablution, the patient stands up, and the servant flings it over his head and body; rub the body well for five minutes, then take off the wet sheet, and put on a dry one. This is a certain relief for fatigue and over-exertion.

COLD WET BANDAGES.

COOLING BANDAGES.—These cold wet bandages are used to produce two diametrically opposite results; to refresh and calm, and to excite and stimulate. Those which are to refresh are for cases of inflammation, congestion of blood, headach, rheumatism, &c.; and with these the sitz-baths are used. To prepare them, linen is first wetted in cold water, then doubled in several folds, and applied to the parts affected. There they must remain until warm; fresh ones are then to be applied; and so on until the complaint be remedied. These bandages should always be accompanied by the sitz-baths, which allay the inflammatory symptoms concomitant on fractures and wounds, and lessen the increase of heat to the head.

FOMENTATIONS, OR STIMULATING BANDAGES—Are of a different nature and effect, but of even greater importance. They are dipped in cold water, and then well wrung out. They must then be applied to the part affected in a manner to exclude the outward air: to effect this, an outside bandage is placed over the first, and the moisture is thus retained and thrown back. Heat is thus generated, and heat of this humid nature has an exciting and dissolving property, which stimulates perspiration and draws out the vicious humours, as can be clearly shown by the bandages and the water they were worked in at Gräefenberg. Mr. Claridge tells a story of a prince, whose name he does not mention, "who, twelve months previous to going there, had rubbed into his leg a light green ointment for about a fortnight, and found that at Gräefenberg the whole of it came out of his flesh by means of these bandages." When become dry, they are taken off and fresh ones applied; but this is not done during the night. They are applied to different parts of the body, and are one of the most important remedies of the cold water system. The ways in which they are worn are numerous. For throat and chest complaints they are worn one round the neck, one on the breast, at night; for weak inflamed eyes, one is worn at the back of the head or neck, at night; for weak digestions and in debilitated cases, one round the waist, all day; and for gout and rheumatism, the legs are wrapped in them night and morning. The *umschlag*, a stimulating bandage, is always used for wounds, bruises, and diseased parts, and generally when pain is felt in any particular region of the body. Its alleviating power is most surprising. The bandage for the waist is a towel three yards long and one foot wide; of this one-third is dry, and two-thirds wetted. The wet part is placed on the belly; the dry covers it, and is furnished with strings which secure it round the body. This stimulating bandage is looked upon as a certain cure for intestine congestion, constipation of the bowels, relaxation, colics, and gripes. It rallies the powers of the stomach, increases the warmth or heat of the stomach, and, by assisting digestion, enables the system to form "better juices." Gout, rheumatism, enlargement of the bones, arthritic concretions, abscess with ulcers and without, chronic, inflammations, and ural chronic complaints of every kind, demand the application of these bandages, and yield to them. Cancers, caries, and syphilitic ulcers, are treated in the same manner. The bandages assuage the pain, calm the symptoms, and what is more, quicker and better than all the ointments and plasters of the pharmacopœia. These bandages promote the swelling of bad humours, and at the same time protect the parts from painful contact with the air. Ointments and plasters, indeed, are vain when compared to these cold wet linen bandages; they are much more easily impregnated with the bad humours. It is vain to attempt to cure malignant ulcers, cherished and nourished in the system by impurity of the blood, with ointments. When were they ever known to purify the blood sufficiently so as to work out a thorough cure? Now, by the system of Hydropathy, as pursued at Gräefenberg, this cleansing process is carried on without difficulty. The ulcer itself acts as a cleanser in exuding the bad humours, the general cure which his going on throughout the body, tending to purify and invigorate the blood, and giving to every process of nature a healthy tendency. Nay, more; if no ulcers existed, this treatment would result in abscesses, which would of themselves spontaneously appear, to serve as channels to carry off the vitiated humours.

THE WET SHEET.—We shall alarm our readers, when we say, in respect to fever, all diseases of the skin, as ringworms, small-pox, measles and scarlet fever, the patients are to be wrapped in a wet sheet! We wonder not at the surprise expressed.—Nothing, however, can be more true, and also more consonant with reason. This kind of fomentation tends to calm and soothe the patient, it assists the eruption, and excites, in fevers, a salutary perspiration. To use the wet sheet properly the following is the process:—Spread a blanket on a bed, then on it a wet sheet, which must have been well rung out; wrap the patient close up in it, except his face; wind the blanket round the body, already cased in the sheet; then add plenty of blankets, tuck them well in, and soon the heat, the perspiration you desire, will have been generated. To stop fever, change the sheet every half-hour. "In desperate cases," says a medical writer, "we have known this done fifty times in twenty-four hours, and perseverance in this treatment ends infallibly in success." As soon as the fever has slackened, the patient, after being let to lie for a time in the wet sheet, to recruit himself and excite perspiration, is placed in a bath of half cold water (about 64° Fahrenheit), for a quarter of an hour; during which time two persons must rub him briskly with the hand, water being taken up from the bath every now and then, and poured over his head and shoulders. If fever comes on, which shows itself by cold shiverings, persevere in the bath, even for hours, until a genial heat overspreads the whole body. If a bath cannot be got conveniently, throw a sheet wetted, but not wrung out, over the invalid, and let it be well rubbed against the body for five minutes. These wet sheets and bandages are not unpleasant long, they get warm almost directly; but we must not regard inconvenience or unpleasantness for a cure. Are drugs, blisters, bleedings and leeches pleasant? do they, *for certainty*, effect a cure? Yet if the latter question were asked of M. Priessnitz's treatment it would be answered in the affirmative. In no case of fever, however violent, has he yet lost a patient! We know, by experience, that the application of cold water relieves the skin, excites it, and disencumbers it of obstructions which close the orifices of the pores; a re-action of the whole system ensues, a heat being created on the surface of nearly fifty degrees above the usual temperature of the body. The part afflicted imbibes a portion of the water, which, in conjunction with the new heat occasioned, softens and dissolves the morbid humours, and assists in their exudation by the pores of the skin. If any doubt be entertained on this subject, all that is necessary is to refer to the fact of the disagreeable colour and smell proceeding from the bandages at Gräefenberg, and which partake of the nature of each particular case. To the uninitiated the notion of applying wet linen to the body, will of course, at first seem one of great danger; the old prejudices against wet clothes and damp linen will immediately revive before them in startling array. How little danger and how much benefit there is in these applications is best proved by the practice of M. Priessnitz, of Gräefenberg, who adopts them as his first steps, with the aged, with infants, with persons of weak and delicate constitutions, and with the nervous; for the purpose of hardening the skin, preparing them to take the bath, and strengthening their system generally, before submitting them to any other application of his cold-water process. As for catching cold through wearing wet bandages at night, such a thing is never heard of amongst the hundreds who at Gräefenberg wear wet bandages through every night. Let but those afflicted with sore throat, or any pain, try them, and they will soon be relieved. The effects of lying in a wet sheet for half an hour are most soothing. Weak patients do so often twice a day, and if children are restless and without sleep, the wrapping of them in a wet sheet will bring immediate relief. The bandage, or *umschlag*, is thus made:—First take a piece of linen, double it in two folds, dip it in cold water (warm will not do), and wring it well out; over this place a dry bandage, sufficiently large to cover the first. This is the whole mystery of this part of the cold-water cure. They are worn together on various members of the body, as they may be affected—mostly by night only, but in cases of pain by day also—and, simple as are these means, their effects have been so wonderful, that of themselves—alone they would suffice to render immortal the name of the peasant Hydropathist—VINCENT PRIESSNITZ.

CÔLD WATER DRINKING.*

The great inventor of the system prescribes only such quantity of water to be drunk as can be taken by the stomach *without inconvenience*. Twelve glasses *per diem* is

* Many object to the drinking of cold water, on the ground that animals only drink to quench their thirst. This is true; but they do not live in our artificial state, nor are they subject to the influence of the mind. It cannot be denied that the nearer people approximate to nature, the less they need adhere to any prescribed rules; but man, recurs to water, to establish his health,

the least that should be drunk; and most individuals swallow from twenty to thirty. Nothing is more easy than to accustom oneself gradually to water-drinking. At first no thirst is felt, and the patient therefore cannot drink it; but like us in drinking wine, thirst comes with the very means taken to allay it; so the desire for more water will be speedily felt by those who drink it. And this arises from the vast quantity of juices carried off by perspiration, which nature feels a desire and a necessity to replace. Much exercise also creates thirst, by causing perspiration. The generality, too, of the processes of the cold-water treatment are stimulating, and generate a greater heat, which necessarily excites thirst. M. Priessnitz declares his opinion, that much of this thirst arises from bad juices in the system, and corroborates this assertion by the fact that, after the clearing out of these juices by his treatment, the thirst always ceases. On first taking to drinking water, some patients feel a sickness, some actually vomit, some have diarrhœa; all which symptoms tend to prove nothing more than that the stomach has within it certain bad humours and acrimonious juices, remnants of old diseases, which the water has set in motion and disturbed. Let the patient, then, so far from leaving off his draughts of water, go on to drink more of it, as a means of ridding his stomach of these foreign humours. Let him persist, then, in his water-draughts, and soon will he find, in increased appetite and restored tone of stomach, the benefits of cold water.

When the stomach is overcharged, cold water must be drunk until vomiting or diarrhœa ensues; and when these come on, the patient must still drink cold water until they stop. How far more agreeable is this prescription of M. Priessnitz than the severe diet and regimen prescribed by doctors when the stomach is overcharged! Our method removes all those impurities from the stomach, which by the doctor's prescription, abstinence, would pass from the stomach only to the blood, and thus render impure the whole system in place of a part. Vomiting by drugs produces the same effect; but how materially does this weaken the system! Cold water, on the contrary, has exactly the contrary effect, of strengthening the organ.

As a beverage, cold water has the most beneficial properties: it cleanses and strengthens the stomach and intestines; it drives out bad juices, and aids in the production of healthful ones; it unites with the blood, being absorbed into it; it diffuses itself quickly through all parts; and liquefying, dissolving, and purifying the acrid and coagulated humours, it finally carries them from the body as perspiration or urine. For trifling indispositions—dyspepsy, and all complaints for which the doctors advise aperient and mineral waters, cold water simply will be found more than efficacious; it restores without weakening the digestive functions. In drinking cold water there can be no danger—in recommending it no quackery; and to those who have an intention of trying at some period the cold water cure at some hydropathic establishment, we recommend the habit of drinking cold water, as it will put the system into a state to facilitate their cure.

TIMES FOR DRINKING COLD WATER.—The best time both for cold water and exercise is before breakfast. At this time they both produce their *best* effects; but the only general rule prescribed by Priessnitz is to drink cold water as much, and at all times, as it can be done without inconvenience. Water may be drunk after breakfast, but the stomach must not be overcharged. At dinner a few glasses may be taken to moisten the food; after that the stomach must be left to itself; and after the lapse of a few hours, we may go on drinking cold water until supper-time. It may be taken after supper, but not so as to disturb the rest. Exercise, which is in itself a part of

therefore the quantity must be increased, not only for the purpose of allaying his thirst, but to dilute, dissolve, purify, and restore, in quantities which must depend upon the inconvenience or pain experienced. By this simple means, serious indispositions are often prevented. Another argument made use of against drinking cold water is, that it produces dropsy. In the first place, it is evident, that if this were true, such a complaint ought not to exist amongst us, for whoever heard of an Englishman drinking too much water? But we affirm, on the contrary, that this disease is caused by the injudicious administration of drugs; the use of too large a quantity of them; by omitting to drink cold water, and by neglecting to wash or bathe the body daily in that element.

If the skin is so much relaxed that it no longer throws out those matters which daily reach it from the interior of the body, fluids are collected underneath the skin which ought to be evaporated, and which cause inflation, paleness, and cold; this is what is called dropsy.

The more the human body is injured by drugs, the more it is in need of strong perspiration, because it endeavours, by the aid of this physical agent, to relieve itself of all diseased matter; from this it may be inferred, that no persons are in more need of the cold water cure than those who have taken too much physic. Further, strong poisons, of whatsoever nature they may be, whether mercury, blue pill, calomel, bark, or spirituous liquors to excess, frequently cause death by dropsy; sometimes this disease is caused by catching cold, but only those are liable to it who have produced a disposition to the complaint by relaxing the skin. The only remedy formerly known was to draw off the water by tapping, which operation, often repeated, gives a respite to life for a short time. This illness, in its infancy, may always be speedily cured by Hydropathy; and, in its most advanced stages, if there be any strength left in the constitution, this disease will be eradicated by the cold water cure; it being the property of this treatment to revive the activity of the skin, and enable the latter to indulge freely in the necessary ejection of perspiration.

From the returns of the year 1841, within the city of London and Bills of Mortality, amongst a people altogether opposed to the use of water, we find that from dropsy alone, the deaths amounted to no less a number than 584. Any one who never takes physic, nor intoxicating liquors, and keeps to a water diet, may be perfectly sure of never being attacked with dropsy.—*Hydropathy, or the Cold water Cure, as practised by Vincent Priessnitz, at Gräfenberg, Silesia, Austria. By* R. T. CLARIDGE, ESQ.

the curative process, excites the beneficial action of the water, and greatly promotes the cure. *The water* should be fresh from the spring, and as cold as possible. Stoppers must be kept in the bottles and decanters which hold it, as the water then will preserve its coldness and freshness much longer.

COLD WATER INJECTIONS.

COLD-WATER CLYSTER.—The first and most generally used of cold-water injections is, the cold-water clysters, which are used generally for constipation of the bowels and diarrhœa. These diseases are opposites, but both proceed from the same cause—weakness of the intestines, which is remedied by giving tone to these organs, and regulating their functions. The object is effected by the use of the cold-water clyster. At first, the intestines being unaccustomed to them, they must not be applied for more than two minutes; but afterwards, when accustomed to them, the clyster will be frequently absorbed like a glass of water in the stomach. A second clyster is applied directly after the first.

NOSE, EAR, AND OTHER INJECTIONS.—Particular syringes are in use for the various parts. Cold-water injection is also the best means to preserve the teeth, by washing the mouth after eating, in the morning and in the evening. For cold in the head, water sniffed up the nostrils is a sure cure. Scrofula in the nostrils of children, a by no means uncommon complaint, is cured by this means.

These are the methods of using cold water internally. We shall now proceed to describe the external processes.

BATHS.

There are many methods of applying cold water externally. The baths are either entire or partial, of which the latter are foot-baths, sitz (or sitting) baths, and half baths; then come eye-baths, ear-baths, &c., applicable only to particular parts or members. Then come the wet sheets (before mentioned), and then the douche and ablutions.

THE ENTIRE OR PUBLIC BATH—at Gräefenberg, as described by an eye-witness, is " about thirty feet in circumference, and sufficiently deep for a man of the ordinary height to plunge into up to his neck. The water is constantly renewed by springs in the mountains, the waters of which are conveyed through pipes into the bath, and escape by an opening for that purpose, so that no impurities may remain; besides which, the bath is emptied and cleaned twice a day: but this remark applies to Gräefenberg only, as at Freiwaldau (a neighbouring town), most of the houses are supplied with private baths, either small or large, for the use of the inmates. We have already shown that the immersion of the body covered with sweat, into cold water, is exempt from danger, provided the organs of perspiration are in a state of repose. The risk which is incurred of catching cold, if, on arriving at a river to bathe, we remain until the body is cold and dry, cannot possibly exist in this case; as we thereby abstract from the body the heat which it requires to produce re-action, and then lose the good effect of bathing. Then if we walk far, or a long distance to the bath, it is requisite to repose a little in order to tranquillise the lungs, after which we must undress quickly and plunge head-foremost into the water; having first wetted the head and chest to prevent the blood mounting to those regions. This precaution is strongly enforced at Gräefenberg. During the bath the head ought to be immersed several times in the water. It is equally useful to keep in movement in the bath, and to rub with the hands any parts afflicted. The skin is thus stimulated, and the sensation of cold abated. People whose chests are affected must exercise moderation in the use of the bath, entering it only by degrees, and not staying in it too long. In general the time for remaining in the bath is governed by the coldness of the water, and the vital heat of the bather; however, no general rule can be adopted with respect to this. At Gräefenberg, where the temperature of the water is from 43° to 50°, no one stays longer in the bath than from six to eight minutes, many only two or three. Priessnitz advises his patients to avoid the second sensation of cold, which is a sort of fever, by leaving the bath before it is felt; by this means the patient will avoid a too powerful re-action, provoked by a great subtraction of heat. This precaution is indispensable at the epoch of the cure, marked by fevers and irruptions. Then a re-action, produced by an immoderate use of the bath or douche, would compel the invalid to keep his bed for some days, without at all accelerating the cure. Persons who undertake to treat themselves by cold water, ought to observe the rules strictly, as they will have no one to give them advice in case of transgression, when medicine would do more harm than good. There is but one thing which they can use or abuse with impunity, and that is drinking water. On leaving the bath, which is found more refreshing than any one can imagine who has not experienced its effects, you are covered with a sheet, over that a cloak is thrown, and thus you go to your room, where the whole body is dried and rubbed; then you must dress quickly, and walk to keep up the warmth. To effect this, by the heat of stoves or beds, would be acting in direct opposition to the treatment. A glass or two of water immediately after the bath, is agreeable, and should not be omitted whilst walking. When irritation is highly excited during the cure, baths should be suspended, as they would augment it.—A general washing of the body, and sitz-baths, are then resorted to. Sweating is also replaced by the envelopment of the body in a damp sheet, the repeating of which operation, together with the sitz-bath, will cause the irritation to cease."

THE HALF BATH—is one of those of the ordinary size, seen in houses; and is made use of when the patient is too weak to use the entire bath, for such length of time as is necessary for him to remain in it, for the purpose of stimulating into action the morbid humours. It is less efficient than the whole bath, and less active in its operation; and being less liable to dangerous influence, is often given to patients on their first arrival at Gräefenberg, to prepare them in a few days for the entire bath; the temperature of the half-bath is 60 deg. Fahrenheit, never under. The water in a half bath should not be more than from three to six inches in depth. If used in place of the entire bath, the attendant pours water upon the patient, or keeps continually wetting his body and head from the water of the bath; but when these baths are used, their effect is less stimulating than the entire bath; then the body is carefully covered, and the bath so closed as that the head only is seen. This is done in cases where the patient is required to remain an hour or two in the bath. M. Priessnitz has been known to keep an invalid in the bath for five or six hours together, and this for several days successively, in order to excite the skin and produce fever from the irritation. A medical man, suffering from atonic gout, was cured by this treatment. Indeed, at Gräefenberg it is not uncommon to see patients sitting thus inclosed in the half bath for several hours, until fever ensues. The CRISIS* of the complaint is thus brought on:—The morbid matter secretes to the skin in the form of abscesses, which break and occasionally discharge themselves in great quantities, sometimes enough to fill several wine glasses. At this period of the disease, the use of the baths is stopped until the humours are discharged, to the great benefit of the whole system, and vastly to the relief of the patient. The half bath is frequently applied after the wet sheet; in such cases, the whole body is also well sprinkled with cold water, and well rubbed in. Whilst still in a state of perspiration, from the wet sheet, the patient should hurry to the bath, throw off his covering, after wetting the head and chest; and the servant must throw a pail of water over his head; and well rub the face and body—this rubbing frequently continues for a quarter of an hour. On coming out of this, the patient must dry and dress himself, and then take exercise in the open air. In fever cases, we first wrap the patient closely up in a wet sheet, changing it as soon as it becomes warm, for another, which is done until the fever has subsided;

* The crisis is a period in the treatment when nature is about to resume her power over the disease, when the latter has been attacked and is struggling to escape. It may be compared to a tiger, which a man is tempting in its lair; for a short or long time depending upon the caprice of the animal, it lies dormant, only occasionally giving signs of existence; when suddenly it rouses, and a violent struggle ensues; the man, however, proves the stronger of the two, and the animal retires worsted in the rencounter. In all future attacks, too, which are even less vigorous than the first, the tiger is defeated, until it finally quits its lair, and flies from its human conqueror. Thus, at least, are old chronic diseases eradicated: in acute cases, the first rencounter very often settles the affair. It is in a crisis that the giant mind, the wonderful genius of M. Priessnitz, are made manifest. Such is the unbounded confidence of the patient in him, that every one ardently desires to pass through this ordeal, it being the sure road to health. It must be here observed, that though this is very often a painful period, the assuaging power of water, the non-necessity for confinement and change of diet, added to the perfect security which every one feels as to the result, render it tolerable; and the stranger is struck by the novelty of hearing people compliment one another on being informed, that they have passed a feverish night, or that rash or boils have broken out on some part of the body. This is, however, soon explained by the knowledge which they acquire at Gräefenberg, that these are some of Nature's means of resuming her wonted empire over the system. In and amongst the various discharges or evacuations which lead to the detection of disease, perspiration is more remarkable by its frequency. This could not escape the observing genius of Priessnitz: and it consequently became one of the chief agents or instruments in his mode of cure. "If we consider," says he, "the quietude of the circulating and respiratory organs when not stimulated by drugs, or agitated by any violent movement of the body or mind, we can easily conceive that cold water drunk during a perspiration caused by the concentration of the natural heat of the body by blankets or other coverings which are brought in immediate contact with the skin, far from deteriorating the constitution, must greatly refresh and relieve it." This is a fact which all invalids who have tried the experiment readily admit. An officer in the Prussian army, author of the most concise and best-written work on the cold water cure, told the author that six years ago he was radically cured at Gräefenberg, of a complication of diseases, to the astonishment of all the medical men whom he had previously consulted: that he had the so-called crisis there: the first crisis was painful and distressing in the extreme, rheumatism returned to each part where he had previously felt it; his foot, which several years before had suffered from being trod upon by a horse, was exceedingly painful, his hands and feet became double their ordinary size, and any one might have tracked his path to the bath by the discharge from the latter. This lasted for about ten days. Afterwards he had two other attacks, each inferior in intensity to the preceding one. After the last he found that his hearing, which he had lost for two years, was perfectly restored; he could walk as well as ever he did, a necessary pleasure of which rheumatism had altogether deprived him: in fact, he was a new man, and since that period he has been perfectly well. This gentleman said, that whilst in a fortress, after his cure, with his regiment, almost all the officers, except himself, suffered from influenza, which he completely escaped, by drinking cold water, and making several ablutions a day. Not only did these means preserve his own health, but he had the great satisfaction of being useful to his aged mother, through their medium. This lady, on awaking one morning, found that she was wholly deprived of the use of one side of her body. As she lived in the country, far from any physician, nothing remained but for the officer to exercise the knowledge he had gained at Gräefenberg, and in this he proceeded as follows:—First, he caused three women to rub her as hard as they could all over, particularly on the side afflicted, with their hands dipped in cold water, for half an hour; then, he had her placed in a wet sheet for about the same time, and from that immersed in a bath with the chill off the water; here the women again rubbed her for fifteen minutes; she was then dressed, and was able to walk about and use her limbs as if nothing had occurred.—*Hydropathy, or the Cold Water Cure as practised by Vincent Priessnitz, at Gräefenberg, in Silesia, Austria. By R. T. CLARIDGE, Esq.*

we then place him in the bath, and set two attendants to rub him well all over with the hand until the symptoms are abated. He then joins, if at Graefenberg, the company in the promenade or at the public tables. At night, if he feels any feverish symptoms, the same process is again gone through, and repeated until he is declared to be cured. No change of diet and no confinement to room is deemed requisite at Gräefenberg under the cold-water treatment.

THE FOOT-BATH—Is used almost solely for the purpose of counteracting the morbific agents operating on the upper part of the body. By the system of M. Priessnitz, these baths are used when the doctors would order warm baths. Thus headachs, toothachs (those which are violent more especially), inflammation of the eyes, and flow of blood to the head, are always treated and relieved by the foot-bath, with the addition of wet bandages on the parts affected. The foot-tub for these baths should not contain more than from two to four inches depth of water—just enough to cover the foot, not the ancles, for toothach an inch is enough, and the time from a quarter to half an hour. For sprains the water must be up to the ancles. The water must be changed as soon as it feels warm. Rub the feet while in the bath to produce re-action. Go into the bath with your feet warm by exercise; and on leaving it, take exercise without delay, to restore to them the warmth. Friction with the hands will promote the desired warmth. Cold in the feet is best prevented by cold foot-baths; warm water weakens the skin, excites the pores, and renders the feet more ready to feel cold. If your feet feel cold, do not run to the fire; exercise will warm them better. To prove the beneficial effects of the foot-bath, and how it preserves us from catching cold, we need only feel our feet two hours after the cold bath. They will be found very hot. Before exposure to excessive cold, as in travelling, it would be well to take a cold water foot-bath two hours before setting out. After travelling or any great fatigue, a cold water foot-bath previous to going to bed, will be found greatly refreshing. In gouty cases advice should be taken before using foot-baths; but to people in general, M. Priessnitz prescribes their general use, as tending to check the frequency of these serious complaints, so many of which, he contends, have their origin in the feet.

HEAD-BATHS.—These are used for rheumatic pains in the head, and rheumatic inflammation of the eyes; for headachs, deafness, and affection of the smell and taste. They set in motion by their action those morbid humours which nature mostly causes to issue from abscesses in the ears. In cases of an influx of blood to the head, they are also used; but their use never extends beyond a few minutes, lest too great a re-action take place. Exercise in a shady place in the open air should be taken immediately after them. The following is the method of using the head-bath:—A rug is laid upon the floor, and at the end of it a basin, with a towel at the bottom of it, on which the head may rest, is placed. The patient lies down on the rug, so that his head may lie upon the basin. The back of the head is first placed in the water; next one side of it, and then the other; and lastly, the back part of the head again. The time for which this bath should be used depends on the complaint. For deafness, affections of the smell or taste, and chronic inflammation of the eyes, the bath is to be taken for an hour; that is, one quarter of an hour for each part separately—the back of the head, the sides, and the back of the head again. When persevered in with firmness, a cure is sure to result from these baths. Violent pains of the head generally precede, which terminate in an abscess, on the breaking of which, and the exudation of the humours, the patient recovers. For common headach, the back of the head may be kept in the bath for a quarter of an hour, and the sides five minutes each: in obstinate cases, a foot-bath and a sitz-bath for half an hour each, the water chilled, may be taken with advantage.

FINGER-BATH.—Used for whitlows. Put the finger in a glass of water four times a day, for a quarter of an hour each time; place the elbow in water twice a day, and put on a heating bandage above the elbow, to draw the inflammation from the hand.

EYE-BATH.—An eye-glass or small glass made for the purpose, of the size of an eye, is filled with water, and held to the eye, which after a minute is opened to bathe in it. The head-bath is used mostly with the eye-bath, though not so often; and in inflammatory cases, a heating bandage is placed at the back of the head on going to bed, and another worn on the back of the neck through the day. Weak eyes are cured by wearing a heating bandage on the forehead at night.

LEG-BATH.—In cases of ulcers, wounds, or rheumatic pains, the legs and thighs are put into a bath: these may continue an hour. They invariably bring out abscesses, and if already existing, cause them to suppurate more freely. This treatment applies also to any part similarly affected.

THE DOUCHE BATH.—Of all remedial means employed in the cold-water treatment of M. Priessnitz, the douche is the most efficacious, in setting in motion the morbid humours and routing them from the parts they have seized upon for years, In long-continued complaints the douche is also a most powerful remedial agent. It removes the weakness of the skin, brought on by the sweating process, and strengthens it. It renders the body hardy, and fortifies it to endure all changes of the air. It powerfully excites the muscular and nervous systems. The following is the account given of the douche at Gräefenberg, and its uses by an eye-witness:—" What is understood by a douche, at Gräefenberg, is a spring of water running out of the mountain, conveyed by pipes into small huts, where it falls from the top in a stream about the thickness of one's wrist, which fall constitutes the difference between the douche and a shower-bath: outside this hut is another for dressing, constructed like the first, in the rudest way imaginable. There are six douches in the forest of Gräefenberg, the fall of the first is fifteen feet; the second, ten feet; the third, twenty feet; the fourth, eighteen feet. The douches set apart for women have a fall of twelve feet each; the diameter of the fall is the same as in those of the men. At the colony, there is a douche which is available all the winter; this is not the case with the others. About half a mile out of the town of Friewaldau, there are four douches more, resorted to by both sexes. Nearly all the douches are at some distance from the places of residence of the patients, which occasions a walk to arrive at them, so that the body is in a glow, and better calculated to be benefited by the effect of the water, when submitted to the process. Parts afflicted should, for the greater part of the time, be exposed to the action of the douche, though it must be received occasionally upon all parts of the body, except on the head and face, unless this is especially ordered by Priessnitz. Weak chests should also avoid it on that part and the abdomen, otherwise the fall of water on the lower part of the stomach or belly is not injurious. The atony of this region will not, however, always resist these means. The relief afforded by the douche, sometimes in a few minutes, in arthritic cases and rheumatism, is almost miraculous. The douche being intended to put the morbid humours in movement, ought to be discontinued when it produces feverish excitement, and be commenced again when that has ceased. The duration of the douche is from three to fifteen minutes, and rarely extends beyond the latter. The time for douching is one hour after breakfast, and two hours after dinner. Most of the patients at Graefenberg are very much pleased with this part of the treatment.

THE SITZ-BATH.—So called from the German word implying a sitting-bath—a bath taken while seated—a small shallow tub of about eighteen inches diameter—the water about three or four inches in depth; the patient sits in this, with his feet rested on the ground, for a quarter of an hour, half an hour, or longer, as may be thought requisite. Sometimes this bath is taken twice or thrice daily. It is very general as a mode of treatment at Gräefenberg. It strengthens the nerves, draws down humours from the head and chest, relieves flatulency, and has the most important results to those who lead a sedentary life. No more water must be used in this bath than three or four inches at the most; as a larger body of water would remain cold, and perhaps cause a congestion to the upper extremities; but, being small in quantity, it quickly becomes of the same heat as the blood, and allows of an instant re-action. A wet bandage to the head will, however, prevent any congestion; while the effect of the sitz-bath may be much advanced by rubbing the abdomen as much as possible, while in the bath, with the wet hand.

A FEW WORDS ON THE EFFECTS OF COLD WATER IN ITS EXTERNAL APPLICATION.

The skin by which the body is covered, far from being merely a protecting envelope, serving mechanically to defend the subjacent parts, is one of the most important organs, the continual activity of whose functions is an essential condition to health. This organ, entirely neglected in our days, has become a source (too little known and appreciated) of most diseases.

As the last ramification of the nerves, which are the organs of sensation, terminates on the surface, the *skin* is the seat of a sense the most powerful and most frequently employed, the touch, or feeling, by which we come in contact with other bodies, and, above all, with atmospheric air. It is, then, principally in the state and constitution of the skin that we must discover the reasons for the different degrees of susceptibility in different diseases, the sensibility of all persons to change of weather and temperature, such as draughts (which are called rheumatic tendencies), and the ease with which so many persons perspire, and are thereby liable to constant colds.

Absorption and exhalation are two other important functions of the skin, which are effected by means of innumerable pores which appear on the surface, where the hairs appear, and on which abut the orifices of numerous vessels that terminate there.

By absorption we introduce into the animal economy all those fine and imperceptible substances, which enter more or less into the composition of the corporeal frame.

Exhalation, or cutaneous perspiration, consists in the perpetual evacuation of substances no longer requisite for the nourishment of the corporeal substance. This insensible, incessant excretion, produces a vaporous liquid, only estimable by its smell and weight, yet so great that, according to exact observations, the skin in a healthy state, without sweating, conveys from the body daily three pounds of used and corrupted substances. As the free exercise of all the excremental secretions must thus be of the greatest importance to health, we can easily imagine the ills that must follow the suppression and derangement of perspiration; in fact, if this cutaneous perspiration be prevented by an obstruction of the pores, the matter of which this excretion would have relieved the body is thrown upon the organic system, and causes all sorts of diseases.

On the other hand, the more active the skin may be, and the more freely the insensible perspiration is carried on, the less have we to fear rheumatisms, catarrhal affections, &c. This will show how it happens, that in a highly dangerous disease, one strong sweating alone is enough to arrest its progress and cure it, since it relieves the system from the unwholesome matter which had caused the disease.

Now, we may ask, is it possible to discover a better plan to preserve the vitality of the skin, and aid a free perspiration, than pure cold water? Our ancestors, who were well convinced of this truth, and put it into practice, enjoyed more vigorous and lasting health than their descendants. What, then, can be more surprising than the fact, that in days, when the cultivation of the mind, of sciences, and of arts are brought to such high perfection, we should still see that important organ, the skin, necessarily demanding such essential care, entirely neglected, and ablutions and cold baths, the true and only means of assisting the action of the cutaneous function, fallen into such desuetude that the famous Dr. Hufeland, more than forty years since, was compelled to complain that the greater number of men had never experienced the salutary effects of cold water during the whole course of their lives, except at their baptism! We certainly are still accustomed to wash our hands and face every day in cold water; but this is all we have preserved of the health-bearing ablutions and baths of our ancestors; these we observe carefully for the sake of cleanliness; but we limit ourselves to this washing alone, and carelessly neglect other important parts of our bodies, as if they never required to be washed and made clean. Covered and swaddled with clothes, in our darkness we do not see that if the corrupt and dirty matter from daily insensible perspiration, or from sensible sweating, is not carefully cleared from the skin by washing it must increase and attach itself to the skin, close the pores, and obstruct the excretion so indispensable to health, and must inevitably, from such evil tendency, at last produce disease. We relax and debilitate the skin, by dressing too warmly during the day, and sleeping on feather-beds at night, or by washing ourselves with warm water.

Let us look to animals. Do we not still wash and cleanse our horses, lead our dogs to a river, and take care that our poultry have plenty of water? But, as to ourselves and our children, an unaccountable blindness seems to deprive us of the beneficial effects of this indispensable element.

We often see our children languish and fall sick; but we never think that too frequently the only cause of this illness is, the obstruction of the pores of the skin, produced by our negligence in not having purified it with cold water. Are such the profits of the boasted cultivation of our mind and of our profound knowledge?

Nor is the use of fresh water confined to cleansing the skin, and assisting the perspiration; its salutary effects reach much further. The first impression of cold water, it is true, when it comes in contact with our bodies, is unpleasant, arising from the absorption of the caloric, the contraction of the capillary vessels, and the sudden rush of blood and humours towards the centre. The first action of cold water is, to cause a sudden sensation of cold, a shivering, a trembling of the limbs, and an oppression of the chest. But the activity of the organs, concentrated inside, begins on the instant a re-action towards the surface, with force sufficient to dissolve the contraction, to restore the heat, and gradually to assist the circulation of the blood and humours, to aid the secretions and excretions, to strengthen the muscles and nerves, and lastly, to refresh, re-animate, and vivify, in a healthful manner, the entire system. What other way, it may be asked, than this is there to guard our bodies from the dangerous influences from without—this body which we so carefully render, from our births, delicate and susceptible of the slightest current of air, and every change of the temperature? What means can be more securely, or more easily employed, to fortify and make robust, than ablutions and cold-baths?

Dr. Hufeland, whom we have before mentioned, in speaking of cold-baths, says, "they not only purify, not only give vitality to the skin, but refresh the body, and enliven the mind. They strengthen and guard it from atmospheric changes, preserving the suppleness of its solid parts, and the flexibility of its articulations; and, in fact, prolonging vigour and youth, and postponing decrepitude and old age."

For these reasons it is, that doctors of every age and experience give their advice with respect to children, to accustom them, from the most tender age, to this salutary element, by washing the head and feet every day with water, not cold but lukewarm, and diminishing daily in heat, until fresh well water may be employed, and occasionally to subject them in winter, and in summer oftener, to cold-baths. These doctors are aware, that there is nothing more proper to make children less sensible to colds, and other dangerous influences—nothing better fitted to ensure the straightness of the limbs, to strengthen and make robust, to protect against all sorts of cutaneous and other diseases, than cold water.

HOW TO TREAT DISEASES BY THE COLD-WATER TREATMENT.

GOUT.—While all other medicines used hitherto for the cure of this complaint, whether in the feet, the hands, or the knees, are essentially hurtful, though productive of momentary relief, bringing on, as medical treatment invariably does, forced evacuations, a derangement of the digestive functions, and a collection and secretion of acid juices, we may, with a clear conscience, from our own knowledge, pronounce that the Cold Water and Sweating Treatment of Vincent Priessnitz, are the only means which result in a final cure. This method expels from the system the vitiated juices, and strengthens the system by *exhilarating*, rallying, and hardening the digestive organs. Eight weeks are sufficient for a radical cure, however violent the disease. To cure Gout requires the use of the whole Cold Water system. First, it is necessary to obtain relief for that irritability of the skin which is so painful a diagnostic of the complaint. This is done by the use of the baths and the sweating process, combined with exercise in the open air. Progressively, all flannel worn next the skin must be laid aside. In summer, this is done on the fifth day; in winter, somewhat later; and, strange as it may seem, always without any discomfort to the patient. When the patient has sufficient strength, he may next submit himself to the douche bath, at first applying the stream to all parts of his body, and afterwards, as he can more easily bear it, to the part affected; that by such brisk application, the morbid humours there collected may be set in motion.

We now come to the perspiration or sweating process, which, in cases of gout, is of the utmost importance. The patient, wrapped in a blanket, must now bind round the inflamed parts the bandages or swathings, renewing them as we shall hereafter describe. It is rarely that more than six weeks pass over in this stage of the treatment, without that stage coming on in the state of the patient, which M. Priessnitz denominates the *crisis* or turning-point of the complaint in gout. When this crisis comes on, the patient is covered with eruptions and boils, and then the douche bath must be used with moderation; the sweating must be milder, and the patient remain a shorter time in the bath. Sometimes the *sitz* (or sitting) bath alone must be used; sometimes the foot-bath only. Should the crisis be very powerful, the bath is often avoided, the wrapping in a wet sheet used instead. The treatment, thus modified, is kept up till a final cure be effected, unless the irritation of the eruption increase to a dangerous height—it must then be suspended, and cold water fomentation, with bandages, day and night, be applied, adding also the *sitz* baths. These will calm and sooth the irritation. During the whole of this treatment, the gouty patient must drink plentifully of cold water to thin the humours and excite perspiration. Exercise also should be taken as much as possible. If this cannot be done, the drinking of cold water and frequent washings in the same, must be most carefully attended to. Gout in the head has been cured by these simple means only. Whether the gout be in the lower or the upper extremities, the foot-bath, if persisted in, will be found extremely effective. The diseased parts must be bandaged, and the baths taken once or twice a day for at least half-an-hour each time. The water in these foot-baths should not be deeper than up to the ankle-joint.

SCIATICA.—This is hip-gout, or gout in the extremities: for this the sitz-baths must be used. Increase of pain may be expected, but relief will follow. The douche bath may also be here used in addition with great advantage—the gouty humours will soon come down to the feet; then use foot-baths and sitz-baths alternately. The *douche* in all gout cases must be strongly applied. The continual application of wet bandages and friction on the part affected, in the cold-bath, dry rubbing when wrapped up in the blanket, must be carefully applied, as these frictions tend to set in motion the arthritic humours.

TIC DOLOUREUX.—This is in itself a species of gout. The douche must not be applied to the head for gouty pains, in which wet bandages, particularly on the temples, are sufficient; foot and sitz-baths being also taken to bring the humours down to the extremities; but in Tic Doloureux the treatment must be somewhat different; and here, we think, we cannot do better than extract what is said on the subject of this complaint, by R. T. Claridge, Esq., the well-known inventor of the asphalte pavement, who was himself a patient of M. Priessnitz, at Gräefenberg, and who has collected several documents from physicians and other patients, and recently published them in a work on "the cold water system." "The first thing," says Mr. Claridge, "is to water the whole of the body with cold water; if these are insufficient, a sitz-bath should be taken for two hours, a great deal of water drank, and from the sitz-bath immediately to the foot-bath. This treatment is often sufficient to put an end to the paroxysm; if, however, it does not cease, place a cold wet bandage round the head, and take exercise in a place where the temperature is cold. The pain got rid of, the patient should keep quiet for some days, and abstain from perspiration; during the days of relaxation, a sitz-bath must be taken one day, and a foot-bath the next, and wet bandages frequently renewed to the afflicted parts, not forgetting to drink plentifully of cold water. It is necessary to take exercise in the open air after each bath. This is the way in which I treated the dreadful nervous Tic Doloureux, which had almost reduced me to despair, and at last triumphed. I must confess that I made a firm resolution to execute all the requisite operations during the advancement of the disease. But what is not a man capable of undergoing who wishes to live?"

And here we think we cannot do better than give the whole account of his own case, as given by this Mr. Claridge, a gentleman of whom it is sufficient to say, that from his acuteness, well-known "knowledge of the world," and general experience, as well as from his strong common sense, natural perception, and distinguished attainments, a few words of even faint commendation from him would go further to convince the reader of the truth and efficiency of such a singular system of medical, or rather non-medical, treatment, than fifty treatises written by the most eminent doctors of medicine on the subject. We find these remarks in his preface to his treatise on "*Hydropathy*," which those who wish for the fullest information in this important discovery in the healing art will do well to take as their manual.

MR. CLARIDGE'S ACCOUNT OF HIS OWN TREATMENT FOR TIC DOLOUREUX BY M. PRIESSNITZ.

The invalid having read the powerful reasonings of the different authors quoted in the following pages, most of whom had ample opportunities of witnessing the wonderful effects of water, which they treat of, during the time they were undergoing a cure themselves, will naturally ask his medical adviser if he knows anything of

Gräefenberg or Hydropathy; the latter will of course answer in the negative. Consequently, if he puts another question as to the propriety of going there, we may easily anticipate the answer; this, in many cases, will decide the patient on bearing his sufferings as well as he can, continuing deleterious drugs, &c.; but the invalid who prefers becoming a pilgrim to the temple of Hygeia, must summon up his courage, and be determined not to listen to any arguments opposed to his going; for I believe I never named my intention of proceeding to Gräefenberg in any society where the Water Cure was totally unknown, but every effort was used, by arguing with me, by intriguing with my family, and by summoning up a whole host of imaginary horrors, to deter me from so doing. But, on the other hand, I never made known my destination to any persons who had been at Gräefenberg themselves, or who knew any one who had been there, that did not strongly approve of my plan, and who did not speak of the astounding success of Priessnitz in his treatment of disease, in the strongest terms that language could express.

Some years ago, a friend of mine at Gratz in Syria, who had received in his own person a most miraculous proof of the efficacy of the treatment at Gräefenberg, strenuously recommended me to go there; but as almost every one is prodigal of advice, and as one every day hears of some vaunted panacea, it made no more than a momentary impression upon me, and was, therefore disregarded. My attention was first seriously drawn to the subject, by a distinguished officer of marines at Venice, who was some years ago so reduced by fever in the East, as to be unable to continue the service in which he was then engaged. M. Priessnitz, whom he met at Vienna, advised him to drink bountifully of cold spring water, and to use it constantly in external ablutions. From that time to the present, he has seldom failed to drink from ten to fourteen glasses of water a day, and bathing in the Adriatic winter and summer; during which period he was unconscious of pain and became strong and robust. Seeing me attacked by rheumatism and head-ach, to both of which complaints I have been subject for the greater part of my life, my friend strongly advised me, in the winter of 1840, to follow his example.

At an evening party at Venice, I was introduced to one of the leading medical men who attended the Imperial court at Vienna, and the British Embassy in that city; on my inquiring of him if he knew anything of Gräefenberg, he told me that as empirics are not permitted to practise in Austria, some years ago, on a complaint being addressed to the Government at Vienna, against M. Preissnitz, the Aulic Council appointed him and two others to proceed to Gräefenberg to inquire into and report upon the truth of the allegations, the danger or utility of the system, &c.; that he proceeded there, as directed, and without entering into details, he would leave me to judge what he thought of it, by the fact, that M. Priessnitz was not only allowed to practise, but was honoured by the friendship of some of the members of the Imperial family.

On asking him if he thought the treatment would be advantageous to me, he replied in the affirmative, and said that he frequently sent his own patients to Gräefenberg.

On arriving at Rome, after being confined to my bed and room at Florence for nearly two months, I endeavoured to induce a friend, who was extremely ill, to accompany me to Gräefenberg; this he would not consent to, without first speaking to his medical adviser, who was a German. Much to the credit of this liberal man, he answered my friend's inquiry by saying, "you are too much reduced for so long a journey at present; or I should advise you to undertake it; for I have been myself at Gräefenberg, and have seen Priessnitz undertake cures, from which any medical man would have shrunk. I fancy he is so completely ignorant of human anatomy, that if asked where the liver was situated, he would be at a loss to say; but that he can cure the liver complaint there is not the slightest doubt. Whilst there," he went on to say, "I witnessed cures of such an extraordinary nature as to lead me to believe that Priessnitz must be acting under divine inspiration." Failing to persuade my friend to go, I nevertheless prevailed upon two of my countrymen to precede me to Gräefenberg. Now, although my mind was fully made up to go there, I confess that my confidence was often shaken by the fears sometimes very forcibly expressed by persons I fell in with by the way; but I always determined on going and judging for myself.

On arriving at the establishment at Gräefenberg, and finding all the rooms engaged, I was compelled to descend to the town of Freiwaldau, at the bottom of the mountain, where strangers are sure of finding accommodation. The arrival of an English carriage and family, probably for the first time, was too important an event not to be immediately known to everybody. Consequently, early the following morning, our countrymen, whom I had persuaded to go; one, a medical man, who had been there two months, the other one month, called upon me to invite my family up to the establishment that day to dinner. These gentlemen, on our meeting, declared that they owed me an eternal debt of gratitude, for having directed their attention to Gräefenberg, adding, "when we came here we were encased in flannel, to which we have said adieu for ever: our appetites are excellent; and, above all, we sleep well, and exercise never tires us. We have now acquired a buoyancy of spirits quite incredible: had any one told us three months ago it was possible to attain it, we should have treated the idea as chimerical." They then expressed an opinion that it was flannel, abstaining from drinking water, and ignorance of its value in ablutions, and not the damps of England, that caused so many to seek health in other climes, to the evident disadvantage of our own country.

At dinner there were between 200 and 300 persons, of all ages and all ranks in society, who, with perhaps half a dozen exceptions, were invalids, a circumstance which no one unacquainted with the fact would have suspected; for I could not help remarking the happy, healthy-looking countenances of all around, and the merry laugh and mirth which burst from every part of the large saloon. On expressing my surprise to the English doctor, he said, " You will find difficulty, no doubt, in believing that there are, to my knowledge, forty or fifty persons here, who, but for Priessnitz, would have been consigned to their tombs, and not have been living here to-day to tell their tales; and that there are, perhaps, twice as many more who, under any other treatment, would have been confined to their beds. On looking at these people, you must bear in mind that they are not on a par with the casual occupants of an hospital; for the majority of them have come here after having consulted all the celebrated doctors within their reach, and tried the mineral waters in Germany in vain; that they are people who only abandoned their medical advisers when it became too apparent that they could receive no assistance from them, or when they could no longer be induced to follow their prescriptions; therefore, the majority of these cases may be considered more advanced and confirmed than the common run of an hospital; that disease is too firmly rooted in their systems to be relieved by the ordinary practice of the faculty, most of them being considered incurable." The doctor added, " if anything could be adduced to show that invalids can live, digest, and become strong without the aid of drugs, it would be the fact, that amongst the large number of people, both here and at Freiwaldau, some of whom have been many months under the treatment, not a grain of medicine has been taken by any one of them since their arrival. Notwithstanding they eat with appetite that, but for the dissolving power of water, would cause them to die of indigestion. As there is no wine, mustard, or pepper on the table, people think no more of such things than if they were not."

One can easily imagine much gaiety and cheerfulness to exist at the public tables of the different Spas, or at other watering-places, as they are devoted to recreation and amusement; but in an hospital, where almost every disease known in Europe is to be found, the existence of such gaiety appears incomprehensible except to those who have been some time at Gräefenberg, and have witnessed the soothing power of water in the alleviation of pain, and the buoyancy of spirits which it promotes, by regulating the digestive powers.

" Look at your neighbour, to the right," said the doctor; " he came here twelve months ago on crutches, having previously been a year in bed. His disease, the gout, being an old hereditary complaint, he is not yet cured; but one thing he will tell you, that though in pain when he first came, it soon ceased, and he has never been confined to his room an hour since, nor did he ever enjoy finer health. Then look at that young lady opposite. From childhood, she had scrofula in her face and neck to such an extent, that she was an object of pity to all who saw her; she has been here nine months; and is now so completely recovered, that she is considered the beauty of the room. That officer near her is suffering from a wound in his leg. At first it withered away until it became no larger than a man's wrist; the surgeons said, nothing but amputation remained. Upon which he came here, and now his limb has resumed its flesh and will shortly be perfectly restored. Yonder female walking with a stick, was brought here six weeks ago in wet sheets. She had been confined to her bed and room, until she lost the use of her limbs, and so became a perfect skeleton; she now walks tolerably well with a stick, and in a fortnight, it is expected, she will do without it."

He then pointed out a child, who had lost the use of his legs from scrofula, but now perfectly recovered. Another person was tormented for years with tic doloureux, who after remaining here a few months, became perfectly cured. There is an officer now recovered from hernia, and there several others from rheumatism. "That gentleman," said he, " is a field-marshal in the Prussian service; eighty-seven years old: he came here on crutches, with the gout, two months ago. He is delighted with the treatment, and now walks about these mountains, with the use only of a stick. He intends staying here through the winter. That lady from Moscow has a child only three years old distorted by a spinal complaint; four months ago, the poor infant could not stand erect, now it plays about, and is as happy as the other children: in six months' time, it will be perfectly cured." In fact, such a number of singular and extraordinary cases were pointed out to me by my friend, whose knowledge of the facts and veracity could be depended upon, that I no longer doubted the astounding accounts I had so frequently heard of the cures effected at Gräefenburg. The saloon was noble and spacious; but as to the dinner and attendance, I thought nothing could be worse; and no barrack in England could be more divested of what is understood by the term comfort (a word not yet introduced into the German language) as regarded the sleeping apartments. I now debated with myself the possibility of all these people being fanatics—fanatics they certainly were in one sense of the word; but were they deceived? No, no,—this could not be; because here were men of all nations, creeds, and professions, of variously constructed minds, and amongst them, several of the medical profession, who had come here to be cured themselves, and to learn the mode of cure. Nothing but the real merit of the system could induce people to suffer the privations to which they were here subjected; and the certainty of their disease being cured, and their constitutions radically restored; this alone induced them to submit to such privations. Having at last made up my mind to become one of Priessnitz's patients, I was prepared for his coming in the morning.

The first thing he did was to request me to strip and go into the large cold-bath, where I remained two or three minutes. On coming out he gave me instructions, which I pursued as follows:—

At four o'clock in the morning, my servant folded me in a large blanket, over which he placed as many things as I could conveniently bear; so that no external air could penetrate. After perspiration commenced, it was allowed to continue for an hour; he then brought a pair of straw shoes, wound the blanket close about my body, and in this state of perspiration I descended to a large cold-bath in which I remained three minutes; then dressed and walked until breakfast, which was composed of milk, bread, butter, and strawberries (the wild strawberry in this country grows in abundance, from the latter end of May until late in October); at ten o'clock I proceeded to the douche, under which I remained four minutes, returned home, and took a sitz and foot-bath, each for fifteen minutes; dined at one o'clock; at four proceeding again to the douche; at seven repeated the sitz and foot-baths; retired to bed at half-past nine, previously having my feet and legs bound up in cold wet bandages. I continued this treatment for three months, and, during that time walked about 1,000 miles. Whilst thus subjected to the treatment, I enjoyed more robust health than I had ever done before; the only visible effect that I experienced, was an eruption on both my legs, but which, on account of the bandages, produced no pain. It is to these bandages, the perspirations, and the baths, that I am indebted for the total departure of my rheumatism.

Whilst thus near Priessnitz, and when consequently I had no fear of the result, by way of experiment, I determined, one thorough wet day, not to change my clothes, which were completely saturated, and in this state I sat until they were completely dry: the consequence was, that in the night I awoke with a distracting head-ach, parched tongue, a slight sore throat, and the next morning felt no appetite, but a general languor of body. By the following detail of this case, the reader will judge how easily a cold of this nature is generally cured by Hydropathy. I laid in the kotz, or blanket, went into the cold-bath as usual, and in the afternoon was enveloped in a wet sheet for an hour, until perspiration commenced, then sat in the half-bath, (not quite cold), and was rubbed all over by two men for twenty minutes; walked out as usual; at night, on going to bed, wore the bandages, or umschlags, on my breast and back of the neck; next day repeated the same, and the third day was perfectly recovered.

My family have all proved the beneficial effects of M. Priessnitz's treatment. The night before our departure, the patients gave their annual ball, in the great room of the establishment, in commemoration of M. Priessnitz's birthday. The whole of the buildings belonging to him were illuminated, both inside and out, at their expense. In this assembly, consisting of about 500 persons, no stranger would have believed, had he been acquainted with the fact, that its members were chiefly composed of invalids. Tears were frequently observed to steal from the eyes of many who blessed the great man for their restoration to health; and I do not know a more touching scene than seeing invalids, who, by his means, had regained the use of their limbs approach him, throw their crutches at his feet, and join in the maze of the waltz. Monarchs might have envied him his feeling on such occasions.

On the day of our departure we had been at Gräefenberg three months, during which time our health was perfectly established; we acquired the habit of living more moderately, of taking more exercise, of drinking more water, and of using it more freely in external ablutions than we were accustomed to; and, I may add, that we have learned how to allay pain, how to ward off disease, and, I hope, how to preserve health. My sojourn at Gräefenberg will ever be matter of self-congratulation to me, and will be amongst my happiest recollections. If I am instrumental in relieving the sufferings of my countrymen; if I succeed in bringing to their notice a system calculated to be of such essential benefit to them; if I can prevail upon them to participate in the happy effects of the treatment which I have myself experienced, my feelings of satisfaction, arising from my residence at Gräefenberg, will be heightened in no ordinary degree.— R. T. CLARIDGE.

RHEUMATISM to be treated in the same way as gout—abundant perspiration, the douche and bandage on the parts affected.

FEVER—NERVOUS AND INFLAMMATORY.—All fevers yield to the use of cold water as fomentations—i.e., the wet sheet and the sitz baths, each being renewed, according as the disease is more or less malignant.

FEVER—INTERMITTENT.—The patient to be placed during a paroxysm in a half-bath for long or short periods, and well rubbed all the time with cold water. The patient must use the sitz-bath, and drink copiously of cold water, until it causes him to vomit, or produces relaxation; a cold wet bandage is placed on the abdomen, for the purpose of producing perspiration. By these simple means is a disease cured, which resists, too often, quinine and all the specifics of the pharmacopœia. Every year some hundreds of patients—soldiers from the fortresses of Prussia, where, in the summer months, this disease is prevalent—have reason to bless the system of Priessnitz for their cure.

DROPSY—in its early stages, only, is curable by perspiration and cold wet bandages to the parts affected.

CANCER.—For this awful complaint, *cold water is a certain cure.* The treatment is the same as for ulcers, with the exception that perspiration is mployed. In cases of Cancer the patient must be made to perspire every day.

CHOLERA.—The constitution of the patient, and the nature of the attack, must be considered in the method of treatment. The water should not be so cold when the constitution is feeble, and the sweating should not be so frequent. If the patient be senseless, cold clysters should be given; if attacked with vomiting and stools, he should be placed in a sitz-bath at sixty-two degrees. In case of headach, apply cold fomentation, rub the abdomen and stomach with as little intermission as possible, and at the same time let another rub the back, arms, and legs, with the hand frequently wetted in cold water; and let this rubbing be kept up until the natural heat comes back to the skin. Copious doses of cold water must be taken in large quantities, as on this depends the cessation of the vomiting and looseness. In this disease most especially are these large draughts of water absolutely essential to the restoration of the patient. As soon as the symptoms relax in power, the invalid should be placed in a bed, and rubbed with a dry hand; and then the sweating process be commenced. As soon as perspiration appears, he is cured. Should the symptoms occur again, the same course must be adopted. When the patient sweats, the windows may be opened as the invalid feels inclined. Next, he should be carried to the bath; and then, if he be sufficiently strong, exercise must be taken, and a bandage kept constantly on the stomach. During the sweating process, cold water must also be drunk in large quantities. If of a weak habit, the patient must be kept quite quiet, as repose is the best restorative of exhausted nature; if, however, the patient be robust, let water quite cold be used, and let the sweating be more frequent. The disease is strong, and must be treated with energy. In the early stages of Cholera the cold water treatment is quickly efficacious; but if too long a time has been suffered to elapse, the cure is not so quick: if persevered in, however, success is sure to crown the effort. Fresh water only should be used in the baths and ablutions; if too cold, a little hot water may be poured in to raise the temperature. To cure cholera, perspiration must be reproduced, and this can only be brought about by restoring vital energy to the skin by the circulating qualities of cold water. To effect this, the water must be kept at an equal temperature, by renewing it as it becomes heated. When placed in the bath, the patient should not be immersed lower than the navel, the thighs and legs being out of water should be strongly rubbed to restore the warmth. As regards the temperature of the water, it can be easily imagined that, were it too cold, it would be dangerous; for, failing immediate reaction, death might follow—to avoid this, let the temperature of the water be proportionate to the remaining strength of the patient; the ablutions which are used only after the sweating process to refresh the heated parts must be of short duration, not longer than three or four minutes. If cramps come on in the extremities, they should be placed in water, and friction applied until the pain ceases. Those attacked with cholera, must eat little, avoid milk, and drink copiously of water. The cold water process must be continued for some time, not only to keep up the strength when once restored, but also to completely root out the evil humours which have caused the disease.

STIFFNESS IN THE JOINTS.—The bath to be used for the diseased parts during two hours, and the douche twice a day. Frequent friction also to be applied. If the complaint be of long standing, the sweating process must be also used. When the crisis of the disease arrives, which generally shows itself in boils or abscesses on the parts affected, the douche should be omitted, and not used again until they have healed. The body must be covered and protected from the water, so that the diseased part only be splashed by the water.

CHILBLAINS.—Heating fomentations or bandages to the parts affected, if recent; if of long standing, the sweating process. The complaint arises from vitiated and stagnant humours.

COLD FEET.—Cold foot-baths to be taken twice a-day, for fifteen or twenty-five minutes, and the feet to be bound up at night in a heating bandage. Exercise to be taken freely, for the purpose of setting the blood in motion, and distributing it equally through all the parts. Perspiration in the feet is cured by the same treatment, with the addition of the sweating process.

INFLAMMATION OF THE CHEST—arises from a congestion of the blood to the lungs, and a consequent stoppage of the whole system of the circulation. We must first attack this disease by freshening the blood, and dissolving the obstruction and stagnation in the parts affected. Cold water must not be used in the first instance, as it might, in that stage, increase the inflammatory tendency. The use of the entire bath would be also dangerous, as likely to send the humours from the surface to the centre, already overcharged with too much blood. Sitz-baths, which refresh the blood, and cause a strong re-action to the lower extremities, taking the blood away from the afflicted organ, are the most certain means of reducing the inflammation. The temperature of the water must be 60° Fahrenheit; it must be renewed every half hour, until the patient feels certain feverish symptoms. The symptoms of this fever are generally trembling of the limbs, chattering of the teeth, &c. Wet cold bandages on the chest must also be used at the same time as the sitz-bath; indeed, the whole chest must be covered with wet bandages, which are to be replaced by others from time to time. The other parts of the body must be kept well covered, and the extremities well rubbed with cold water by the hands, and while the patient is in the sitz-bath. As soon as warmth is perceived in the hands and feet of the invalid, we may then judge that the universal mass of blood is refreshed, and a healthy circulation recommenced. Next place the patient in bed, wrapping him up in a wet sheet, which will create an irritation, conducing to a still greater circulation; and while in bed let the chest be covered with a cold wet bandage, to strengthen that part of the body. In cases of obstinate disease, the wet sheet and bandages must be sometimes used again. Every time this is done, be careful to wash the patient with water with the chill off. The patient must also, during the whole treatment, drink cold water, but not in large quantities. By this process inflammation of the chest is invariably cured in a few days.

SCROFULAR RICKETS.—If the limbs are distorted, the water treatment will not restore them. The douche bath is principally used in scrofular cases and rickets, and the sweating process is also very strongly applied. The cold water to be used twice each day, and friction applied to the joints and glands (if swollen); bandages, also, are to be constantly employed. Gargling of the glands of the throat and the nose to be also largely used.

SMALL-POX, MEASLES, SCARLATINA.—It is the fever concomitant on these diseases, in which alone there exists danger. As soon as it comes on, wrap the patient in a wet sheet, and let him continue in it day and night. If the fever is violent, another wet sheet must be put on when the first is warm. When perspiration comes on, the patient to be washed in water of 60° Fahrenheit. This treatment will effectually moderate the fever, and the heat which accompanies it. It is the violence of the fever which closes the pores, and the application of the wet sheet moderates the fever, opens the pores, and facilitates the eruption.

ERYSIPELAS.—This is an effort of nature to throw out from the system a humour which obstructs its internal workings. Cold ablutions would, in this instance, have a dangerous tendency to drive in the eruption. The patient must be made to sweat in a wet sheet. Heating bandages are to be applied to the diseased parts. This treatment never fails of success.

HOOPING-COUGH.—The fever of children, as we have before said, is best remedied by the fomentation of the wet sheet. In cases of hooping-cough, this remedy does not so quickly allay the irritation, though it much relieves it. The water given to the child to drink must be tepid, at first, and afterwards must have been at least half an hour away from the spring.

INFLAMMATION OF THE BRAIN.—This is a disease unfortunately too common with infant children, though rare with adults. It is to be treated, whether proceeding from internal disease or external causes, such as a blow or fall, precisely as inflammation of the chest, except that the cold fomentations on the head be frequently renewed, and the wet sheet in which the patient is wrapped, sometimes every ten minutes. If the patient get worse, the sitz bath and the wet sheet must be taken alternately.

INFLAMMATION OF THE EYES—OPHTHALMIA—Proceeds generally from catarrh or rheumatism, and requires to be treated as rheumatism or gout. To the rheumatic process, the eye-bath and the douche are added, in cases of ophthalmia and inflammation of the eye, by M. Priessnitz. The water from the douche bath must be received in the hand, and dashed thence on the eye. Head baths are essential, as also are fomentations to the eyes.

WEAKNESS AND PAIN IN THE EYES.—Baths to the back of the head, a wet bandage over the eyes, worn day and night, eye-baths, and foot-baths soon conquer these complaints. The bandages act by removing the heat from the part affected.

WORM AND RINGWORM.—These foul diseases yield more quickly to cold water than medicines. Sweating in a wet sheet is the invariable process; but ringworm is frequently harder to cure than itch; more time is necessary, and much more cold water vigorously applied. In ringworm, also, the douche must be frequently used to bring the morbid humours to the surface. Ringworm is most difficult to cure when it has been driven in by bad treatment. The disease is altogether of a most obstinate nature, and not easily eradicated, re-uppearing frequently upon the skin after disappearing, apparently under the effects of the douche: a strict attention to diet is absolutely necessary. Mr. Claridge, in his work, quotes (we believe from Dr. Mundé's account, the following cases of ringworm at Gräefenberg:—" Three men, attacked with this disease, arrived at Gräefenberg at the same time as myself; the first of these, after several years' trial of the principal mineral waters recommended in this disease, which he had employed without success. Having followed the treatment with energy for two months, he returned home resolved to continue the treatment mildly all through the winter; after which, he was to come again to Gräefenberg, to finish the cure. At the time of his departure, he was more than half cured. The two others remained at Gräefenberg, one for eight months, the other six, both leaving it radically cured. The treatment of one of these was attended by an acidity rising in the throat, and by the vomiting of matter containing chalky substances. The acidity of the throat was such, that it caused the tongue to be ulcerated. Both, after following the treatment some weeks, saw their ringworms re-appear with greater malignity and more abundant suppuration, attended by the formation of a great number of boils. Following these two cures with great attention, I was not surprised that Priessnitz insisted upon the use of the strong douches, which he directed to be applied to the hips of one of these invalids; he wished a ringworm to appear that had been there formerly. After a time, it again showed itself, spreading as far as the knee, and looking very bad. It is but a few days since I received letters informing me that both the ringworms were radically cured."

MERCURIAL DISEASES.—How dreadful are the diseases arising from the too frequent use of that poisonous mineral medicine, mercury, by the doctors! In the cold-water treatment alone can the invalid hope for a cure; for no method yet discovered has proved so formidable an antagonist to mercury.

MERCURIAL ULCERS.—Treat with the bandages and sweating process. Sweating is the secret. The older the disease the more need for sweating. Purge the blood of foreign humours, and the ulcers will heal of themselves. At first the ulcers will enlarge under the bandages; should this go too far, then dry bandages to be used, and the wounds to be bathed in lukewarm water.

SYPHILIS.—At Gräefenberg, M. Priessnitz, by the sweating process, made a certain, speedy, and safe cure of all cases of syphilis. "I have seen it," says Dr. Mundé, as quoted by Mr. Claridge, "treated and cured with more or less promptitude, according to the virulence, complication, and long-standing of the disease." But first, before proceeding to a cure, it is requisite to eradicate the effects of the mercury, which too many patients have swallowed previous to their arrival at Gräefenberg. Medicine boasts of its cures of syphilis: how many of these said to be cured have had returns of the same symptoms! Whatever be the nature or symptoms of the disease—gonorrhœa, ulcers, chancres, buboes, &c.—the cold-water treatment exhibited at Gräefenberg is the same; viz. sweating, bathing, douching, bandages, and cold water. In cases of gonorrhœa with a discharge, a cold bandage is kept round the part affected, and cold water injected frequently each day. The sitz-bath for an hour or two twice a day, and great attention to diet, soon effect a cure; all nourishment taken must be cold.

THE GRIPES, CATARRH, AND COLD IN THE HEAD.—Perspire in a wet sheet, and wash the body with milk-warm water to assist perspiration. Cold water must be drank plentifully in bed. For inward and external pains, the sitz-bath not quite cold, twice a day for an hour each time; friction must be applied to the abdomen all the time; cold clysters once or twice a day, and a heated bandage round the waist complete the cure.

SORE THROAT, STIFF NECK, COMMON COUGH.—Throat and chest to be well rubbed by the hand dipped in cold water, gargle the throat often with cold water; a heating bandage to be worn round the head and chest.

QUINSY, INFLAMED SORE THROAT.—Bandages of very cold water round the throat, gargles of cold water and frequent sweatings. If strong feverish symptoms be superadded, place the patient in the wet sheet.

EPILEPSY—Is relieved, but not cured, by cold baths and cold water, drank copiously.

DIARRHŒA.—If recent, draughts of cold water, a wet bandage worn on the stomach, and digestible food, will suffice to cure. Diarrhœa is sometimes only an effort of nature to carry off acrid humours, but when chronic it is very weakening; here the sitz-baths are remarkably effectual, they must be taken three or four times a day for half an hour each time. Cold water must be drunk copiously; use cold-water injections, eat moderately, take but little exercise, or rather, if possible, keep in bed. Cold water used for a length of time, will restore proper tone to the organs of the abdomen.

PILES.—This disease, as all know, arises from an overcharging with blood of the vessels which keep moist the lower intestine. They either emit blood, or are dried up and hard by the swelling of the veins. There is a third kind of piles, which emits an offensive humour. This is not merely local complaint; it is rather a demonstration made by nature, to show that the whole system is diseased, and this she expresses by a congestion of the blood at the abdomen. To cure this complaint, a strict regimen is necessary; all heating food, spices, and spirituous liquors, must be avoided. The cleansing and strengthening treatment, therefore, of the cold water cure, is a specific for the piles. If taken in its early stage, the disease quickly yields to regimen, copious draughts of cold water, fomentations on the lower region of the stomach, sitz-baths, and moderate sweating. If the piles, however, are running, the system adopted must be more severe and protracted. Baths, sitz-baths and the douche, will, in the end, effect a cure. Sweating must be resorted to, to drive out the humours which cause the disease. Cold water, outwardly applied, without the sweating, would be likely to prove more injurious; and, by leaving the humours in the system, would, in all probability, change the disease into one more serious. "At Gräefenberg," says Dr. Mundé, "I have seen blind piles open and disappear by degrees, leaving the body in a perfectly healthy state. I appeal to those troubled with piles, of what use are medicinal remedies? A little relief, and never a cure. Doctors themselves are forced to admit this. Several of them, aware of what is going on at Gräefenberg, recommend, and use themselves, the cold-water cure for this disease.

SORE EYES.—A head-bath of cold water to be used for the back of the head only, three times a day, for ten minutes each time. An eye-bath twice a day, for five minutes. The eyes are to be opened in the water. A heating bandage to be worn on the back of the neck at night; the use of which, and of the head-bath, is to draw the humours from the part. The employment of the foot-bath will also be found of advantage in these cases.

ACCOUCHEMENT.—On this important subject we shall quote the words of Dr. Mundé, as corroborated by Mr. Claridge, in his work on Hydropathy:—"Experience has demonstrated the utility of cold ablutions and exercise in the plain air, to females who are *enciente*; to this ought to be added simple diet, and the drinking plentifully of cold water: wine, coffee, and liquors should be avoided. Madame

Priessnitz is accustomed, during the six weeks previous to her accouchement, to take a cold-bath every day. To this she owes the happiness of a prompt and easy accouchement, and her speedy establishment in health."

COLICS—Are cured by sitz-baths, bandages on the abdomen, clysters, and cold-water drinkings. Rheumatic colics are treated in the same manner.

WOUNDS.—The part to be kept in tepid water until the bleeding stops; then a heating bandage to be applied; when this is warm, put a larger one over it. In wounds of the foot, keep the part in the foot-bath twice a day, to draw out the inflammation. The bandage to be kept on night and day, and it must extend beyond the wounded part.

BURNS.—Cold wet cloths to be applied.

WEAKNESS OF DIGESTION—DEBILITY OF THE STOMACH.—The first means towards a cure is to avoid the original causes of the complaint. Let sobriety be observed in place of intemperance; simple food taken instead of artificial. Let the regular meals be limited in quantity; food and drink cold, not hot. Avoid spirituous liquors; breakfast and sup on cold milk. Let dinner consist merely of meat and vegetables. Wear light clothing, and keep an easy mind. Take much exercise, wash often with cold water, and drink plenteously of the spring. Having set these rules to yourself and determined to follow them, let us now proceed to remedial measures. A stimulating fomentation, to cover the lower part of the stomach, must first be worn. A light sweat and a cold bath to be taken in the morning; in the evening, a sitz-bath; and during all these the abdomen and lower stomach to be rubbed with wet hands. The douche, if it can be got, may be used, but not on the stomach; if it cannot be got, let the body be well sprinkled with cold water, beginning on the shoulders, and gradually going down to the abdomen. Let cold water be drunk plentifully, not too much, however, at a time, at meals especially. Before breakfast is the best time for cold-water drinking. Much exercise is requisite in the morning; that in the evening must be more moderate. Great heat should be avoided. "I saw," says Dr. Mundé, as translated by Mr. Claridge, "an invalid arrive at Griæfenberg, who had taken a considerable quantity of mercury; he had for several years felt pains in the stomach, accompanied by violent headachs; each returned every twelve hours, and deprived him of all his faculties, more particularly his digestion. He had tried medicine in vain, without obtaining the slightest relief. He was completely cured at Griæfenberg, not only of his pains, and his bad digestion restored, but his system was purified by sweating out the mercury with which it was saturated, which, no doubt, was the origin of his disease." His treatment was what we have described.

DYSPEPSIA, INDIGESTION, CONSTIPATION, AND DISORDERED BOWELS.—Costiveness is a general complaint, and often goes on till it becomes a disease. Many things cause it: a sedentary life; the habit of stooping at a desk; a hardened liver; weakness or atony of the intestinal canal; and the habit, it must be added, of drinking too little water. Now for the cure. Exercise; the drinking plentifully of cold water; a wet bandage worn on the abdomen; and two or three clysters every day, one upon the other immediately, if it appears necessary. The food must be eaten cold, not warm; fruit also must be largely indulged in; and nothing heavy, or of an oily, greasy nature to be taken. If the costiveness has been of long-standing—say two or three years—sitz-baths and foot-baths must be used. The douche on the abdomen (but with care) corrects any weakness in this part.

SPRAINS, AND STIFFNESS IN THE JOINTS.—In cases of sprains, use the foot-bath, not cold, but tepid, three times a day for half an hour. Rub the sprain well; wear a cold bandage on it day and night. In sprains of the wrist or the hand, use an elbow-bath, and bandage the arm as high as the shoulder. Remember that the bandage should invariably extend beyond the part injured.

HEARTBURN—Arises from over-eating, or from taking food difficult of digestion, or from sedentary habits. To cure it, drink water early in the morning until you bring on sickness or diarrhœa, then away goes the disease, unless of old standing; if so, it is a chronic complaint, and may be attacked accordingly by sweatings, baths, and ablutions.

DEAFNESS.—Friction twice a day over all the body, with a cold wet cloth. A wet bandage over the ears at night. Plenty of water to be drunk. In cases of obstinate deafness the whole hydropathic process must be gone through.

NERVOUS WEAKNESS.—Every one knows that medicine avails but little in this complaint. At Griæfenberg, by the cold water treatment, it is cured with certainty and quickness. Dr. Mundé instances the following cases :—"A lieutenant had his nerves in so great a state of irritation, that the least noise, the barking of a dog, the firing off a pistol, would cause such a headach that he would faint. To relieve this, he had accustomed himself to warm foot-baths. Tired of suffering, he came to Griæfenberg, perspired a little, took every day two cold baths, besides head-baths and sitz-baths, as revulsive measures. This treatment was limited to three weeks, after which he continued his journey. He intended following up the cure at home: Priessnitz approved of his resolution, and advised him to walk a great deal; to ascend the hills, to ride often on horseback, in order to fortify himself also to be enabled to bear fatigue."
"Another invalid came to Griæfenberg with trembling in the upper part of the body, brought on by the excessive use of spirituous liquors. He returned home, radically cured, after two months' treatment; the change from wine to water was not followed by any accident."

Loss of Sleep.—Moderation at meals, and plenty of exercise in the open air, are the best remedies for this complaint. Washing in cold water when going to bed, is more efficacious than the baths. In children sleeplessness is cured by wrapping them in the wet sheet.

Pleurisy, Stitch in the Side.—Foot-baths and fomentation on the part affected will be sure to cure.

Ear-Ach.—Wet bandages to the ears, and linen well wetted with cold water to be put in them; a wet bandage also round the head. If the disease is obstinate, the sweating process and the cold water must be resorted to; in other cases treat generally as for inflammation of the eyes.

Congestion of Blood, Blood to the Head, &c.—These generally affect the head after meals, or after indulgence in wines and heating liquors; also after extraordinary excitement. If subject to this, leave off stimulating foods and drink, eat sparingly, drink water at table; after meals take some slight exercise; avoid all excitement, political, literary, or commercial; and do no business after dinner: to this add the use of cold water as a constant drink; also sitz-baths and clysters, remaining in the baths from half an hour to an hour. Cold wet bandages must be applied to the head, and frequently repeated, to excite the sluggish vessels and give tone to the debilitated organ. A foot-bath and cold bandages are often enough to cure this complaint; the sweating process is avoided, as tending to excite the flow of blood to the head.

Bleeding at the Nose.—Wash the throat and back of the neck with cold water, apply a cold wet bandage to the stomach; take cold foot-baths; if requisite the sitz-bath may be used, and the body may be washed with cold water. A wet bandage placed on the genitals, will frequently check a bleeding at the nose.

Fractures.—Whether before or after the fracture is reduced, cold water is the best means to keep down inflammation. Apply a cold wet bandage to the part; let this remain on one hour, then apply a larger bandage, which will carry off the inflammation from the part. Thus, if the wound is in the leg, the bandage must extend up the thigh.

Inflammation of the Abdomen.—On the instant of the attack, take a sitz-bath of tepid water, and remain in it more or less time according to the symptoms. When coming out of the bath, apply a cold bandage to the stomach, and let the patient be wrapped in a wet sheet. These must be changed every two hours. Each time on coming out of the bath, the patient must be washed all over with cold water. Cold water must be drunk copiously. In cases of women and children, the water must be not quite cold.

Pain in the Chest.—If rheumatic, to be treated like gout. Use friction with a wet hand, and wear a wet bandage at night from the neck to the stomach.

Hypochondria, Hysterics.—This being a disease of the mind as well as of the body, requires fine air, pleasant situation, cheerful society, and a thorough alteration in the plan of living. The uncertain appetite of hypochondriacs is remarkable—now they will eat much, now little, and this irregularity is one of the aggravating symptoms of the disease. For this M. Priessnitz advises copious draughts of cold water, that less space may be left for food.

Tooth-Ach.—The cold water cure for this painful complaint is most simple and efficacious. Take two basins of water; one tepid, the other cold. Fill the mouth with the tepid water, and hold it there until warm; then change it. Meanwhile, dip the hands in the basin of cold water, and rub energetically the whole of the face, the cheeks, and behind the ears. Do this until the pain ceases. The gums may also be rubbed even till they bleed. This is an infallible cure for the tooth-ach. The foot-bath, not higher than the ankles, may also be used with advantage.

Headachs.—These are cured by hot water and head-baths of twenty minutes' duration. For the first ten minutes the back of the head and then the sides, the latter five minutes each, are to be placed in the bath; next the head is to be bound in a wet bandage. Much water must be drunk, and exercise taken in the open air. If the headachs return, the sweating and the cold ablutions must be resorted to. For sweating, the wet sheet is to be preferred, as it assuages the pain.

Tic-Douloureux—Is of two kinds: one purely nervous, which is incurable; the other arising from acrid humours, which at Gräfenberg is cured. Dr. Munde was cured of this complaint in eight months, and Mr. Claridge's statement of his own cure from this dreadful malady has been already mentioned.

Spitting of Blood from the Stomach, Sickness.—This frequently occurs to those who suffer from piles, and nature sometimes acts to repress congestion in this way, instead of by the piles. Sitz-baths to be taken, and cold bandages worn on the chest at night; avoid all irritation of mind and body; seek repose, both mental and corporeal; drink plentifully of cold water. A bleeding from the lungs (as in pulmonary consumption) is not curable by cold water. Of course, the treatment mentioned above is useless, if not followed out by great sobriety and an abstinence from all heating drinks.

Drowsiness—Proceeds frequently from bad digestion, superinduced by overcharging the stomach. In this case the remedy is abstemiousness in eating and drinking. On the first symptom of drowsiness arising from overcharged system, place a cold bandage on the abdominal region, give two clysters of cold water daily, and cause your patient to drink much cold water in the morning, especially before breakfast. Baths, ablutions of the body, and head-baths, should also be applied; and after these, the head must be vigorously rubbed dry. Head-bath and friction to be repeated on going to bed. Exercise to be taken after meals, in order to prevent sleepiness.

UTERINE HEMORRHAGE.—Apply cold water to the abdomen, and if not sufficient, inject cold water into the matrix; the patient must drink plentifully of cold water.

IRREGULARITY OF MENSTRUATION.—Gentle sweatings, general cold ablutions, sitz-baths, and foot-baths, with plenty of exercise and draughts of cold water, scon cure this complaint. From Gräefenberg the ladies go away cured, by hundreds every year.

THE WHITES.—Sitz-baths alone will sometimes cure this complaint; but in general the cold-bath and cold-water ablutions are necessary. Exercise is highly important to the restoration of the functions to a healthy state.

NAUSEA AND SICKNESS.—If merely temporary, drink cold water until they disappear; if a regular disease of the stomach, you must undergo the whole hydropathic process; sweating and half-baths are of essential service.

INSTANCES OF CURES FROM THE COLD WATER TREATMENT.

The hydropathic treatment is distinguished from that of all other medical systems, by its simplicity, its cheapness, and the absence of all mystery in its action and operations; to hundreds of persons at one time and at one place (Gräefenberg) is it administered; and all these individuals congregated together, meet at the same table, and communicate with each other daily, so that whatever of importance occurs to one individual, is known to all and discussed by all; while in all other systems, the patients being attended at home, and invariably kept in ignorance of their own complaint, none but their families or friends can know the progress of the disease and results of the treatment. Let us hear what is said of the great inventor of Hydropathy, M. Priessnitz, by Mr. R. T. Claridge:—

" After the eminent services which this great man, with such modesty and without the slightest pretension, has rendered to society, we cannot be surprised at his having succeeded in securing general esteem. This has been shown by crowned heads and by nobles of the adjoining countries." At present, in 1841, says Mr. Claridge, there are under his treatment at Gräefenberg and Freiwaldau, an archduchess, ten princes and princesses, at least 100 counts and barons, military men of all grades, several medical men, professors, advocates, &c., in all about 500; and the following is a list which shows the progress of the establishment up to the present time:—

1829	45	1837	570
1830	54	1838	800
1831	62	1839	1,400 and upwards.
1832	118	1840	1,756
1833	206	1841, say	1,400
1834	256		
1835	342		7,298
1836	469		

In consequence of similar establishments having sprung up in Russia, Poland, Hungary, Moldavia, Wallachia, and in most states of Germany, it is expected that the numbers of this year, 1841, will not be equal to those of the last; up to the beginning of September, there had been about 1,150. It may not be uninteresting to see how the 1,576 of last year were composed; as by it we may infer that, as the distances in most instances were great, the patients were of the better order of society. It must be observed, that the trades-people or peasantry to whom M. Priessnitz may have given advice, are not included in this list.

	Kurgäste, or "Guests of the Cure in 1840."		Kurgäste, or "Guests of the Cure in 1840."
From Austria	367	From Belgium	7
— Galicia	93	— Italy	3
— Poland	128	— Hamburgh	30
— Hungary	137	— Moldavia and Wallachia	27
— Prussia	527	— Hanover	4
— Saxony	21	— Switzerland	6
— Bavaria	13	— Cracovie	25
— Wurtemburg	15	— Denmark	12
— Duchy of Baden	3	— Brunswick	5
— England	2	— America	12
— Mecklenburg	13	— Other Countries	12
— Sweden	7		
— Russia	94	In all	1,576
— France	15		

On ascending to Gräefenberg by the carriage road, the traveller will see a fountain erected by Wallachian and Moldavian patients, with this inscription:—

" V. P.
" Au Génie de l'Eau Froide."

And on descending by the foot-path to Freiwaldau, he will find another monument of a lion, on a pedestal, in bronze, erected by the Hungarians, with the following inscriptions in their language:—

FRONT.

"As a punishment to man for his presumption in despising the beverage which he had in common with wild animals, he became diseased, infirm, and debilitated.

"Priessnitz causes the primitive virtues of water to be again known, and by it infuses fresh vigour into the human race.

SIDE.

"Priessnitz, the benefactor of mankind, merits the grateful and honourable remembrance of the Hungarian nation; the erectors of this monument invite their countrymen of future ages to the vivifying springs at Gräefenberg.

"MDCCCXXXIX et XL."

Besides what has been done in other states, upwards of forty hydropathic establishments have sprung up in different parts of Germany. There is hardly a journal published in that country that has not taken some notice of this mode of treating disease; and books have been published on the subject in almost every Continental language. England alone forms an exception, which it is difficult to account for. And these enormous results, this wonderful revolution in the medical world, as I may well call it, have all been attained by the zeal, vigour, and genius of one man, and that man originally an uneducated peasant.

Such is the account given by Mr. Claridge; and when we learn that *all* M. Priessnitz's patients are cured, surely it is high time that such a system was brought under the notice of our countrymen.

M. Priessnitz possesses a singular talent in discovering disease, without feeling the pulse or looking at the tongue, or, in fact, resorting to any of the methods adopted by medical men; nor is it every individual presenting himself, nor every complaint, that M. Priessnitz considers curable by Hydropathy, as will be found in some of the following instances:—

INFLUENZA.—A lady for some time had been so seriously affected with pain in the gums, that she could not sleep, and whenever she took cold was confined with pains in the chest. On first commencing under the treatment, she got very feverish and weak, and had the lower part of her face break out into a boil. Her friends remonstrated with her husband on the danger of allowing her to continue under the treatment, assuring him that her chest was affected. Urged by their fears, this gentleman called the attention of M. Priessnitz to them, and seriously requested him to give them due consideration. "Oh," replied M. Priessnitz, instantly, "such fears are groundless; but to ease your mind, I will go and see her." Forthwith he went; and, after a few minutes' conversation, pronounced, without feeling her pulse or asking any questions, her chest quite unaffected; but said she had some complaint settled between the chest and the throat, which, and the pains with it, would be carried off through the boil on the face. The recollection occurred to the lady's friends immediately that she had been long ill with influenza, which corroborated what was said by M. Priessnitz. She soon grew stouter, and her health was thoroughly restored.

CONSUMPTIVE TENDENCY.—A lady and her daughter, on arriving at Gräefenberg, informed M. Priessnitz that the doctors had declared the young lady to be in a consumption. He immediately desired the young lady to run a little way up the hill; when she came down to him, he told her, "There is no consumption, but the system is much that way inclined." The cold-water treatment was then applied. The young lady improved in health quickly, soon grew stout and robust, and in a few months went home completely cured.

TYPHUS.—A Colonel's daughter, who had visited all the doctors and mineral spas of Germany in a fruitless search of health, came at last to Gräefenberg; the crisis of her disorder came on in due course, which from its terrible appearance so alarmed her mother, that with long watching and anxiety, she fell into a low typhus fever. Mother and daughter were now put both under the same treatment at the same time, and both recovered better health than they had ever enjoyed before in their whole lives.

DEAFNESS.—The Colonel himself, hearing this, obtained immediate leave of absence; and though seventy years of age, hastened to Gräefenberg, hoping that a miracle might be worked even then to cure an inveterate deafness of thirty years' duration. He had several other little ailments incident to old age, good living, and the customary inattention to general health, which the usual treatment of M. Priessnitz soon remedied, and the old colonel was delighted at the new vigour and buoyant spirits which were restored to him. One day, sitting in the woods, he thought he could hear the leaves rustle and the birds sing; starting up with great joy, he hastened to M. Priessnitz, and told him he had got back his hearing. M. Priessnitz smiled, and told him "Nothing is impossible to nature, diet, and cold water; but do not be too sanguine, Colonel, your hearing will not last long at present:" and this the colonel found was true; for, to his great vexation, next day he was as deaf as ever. On another, day, however, he caught the sensation of hearing the knives and forks clattering and the buz of general conversation, so loud as to be unendurable; upon this, he again congratulated himself as restored to hearing. M. Priessnitz, however, again assured him of the contrary, which, to his infinite mortification, the veteran found to be again correct. M. Priessnitz wished him to stay three months longer; but the colonel being compelled to return to his post, did so; and adopting the Gräefenberg treatment at his own house, was restored to the full enjoyment of the sense of hearing, at the time specified by M. Priessnitz.

RHEUMATISM.—A German Prince lost the use of all his limbs. After two months' treatment at Gräefenberg, his pains disappeared, his complaint left him, nor has it ever shown itself since.

LOSS OF USE OF LIMBS.—From a dreadful cold, a poor man had lost the use of his limbs. After four weeks at Gräfenberg, his strength was in a great measure restored; and after six weeks, he was walking about and enjoying exercise like the other patients.—A Polish lady of rank had lost the use of her feet and hands through gout and a variety of disorders. Her complaint was so extremely bad, that M. Priessnitz at first declined receiving her at his establishment; but as she obstinately declared she would not go home, but would stop and die at the nearest village to Graefenberg, he was at last obliged to yield, saying he would try what he could do for her case. After the usual treatment for six weeks, he continually inquired if she did not feel pains in the back. At first there were indeed no pains; but in the course of another week they came on strongly, and a large boil broke out in the back. This broke, and she, who had not been able to hold a pen or move a hand for eight years, was now able to write a long letter to her husband, and gradually mended in health.

GOUT IN THE HANDS AND FEET.—A gentleman of sixty years of age, who for several years had been obliged to keep his bed, after six months' stay at Gräfenberg found himself so much better that he returned home, and now treats himself hydropathically at home. For two years he has never been obliged to remain in doors, and finds that his hands and feet are getting back to their original size and shape. This was so bad a case that it may be truly said no victim to the gout was ever a greater martyr than this individual, who now blesses M. Priessnitz and the cold water cure for his restoration to the enjoyment of an existence otherwise almost insupportable.

BLINDNESS.—A Hungarian nobleman of strong frame, was nevertheless of general bad health, and his eyes were so badly affected, that though on looking at them, there seemed to be nothing the matter; yet so grievous was the affliction, that there were but slight hopes of saving them. When he came to Gräefenberg, a friend of his pointed him out to M. Priessnitz, and commenced telling him of his various complaints, amongst others, about his eyes, when turning about and gazing on the baron, who was standing at about four yards distance, M. Priessnitz said, "One eye has already gone, the other can be cured." The treatment of the case went on, and shortly the baron was perfectly blind. He lost all hope, and said to M. Priessnitz, who visited him in his chamber, "Alas! for me the world has lost all its charms, I shall never again gaze on the sweet face of nature!" "No, baron, not so; be comforted :" said M. Priessnitz. "You will see in two days with the other eye. Your sight will grow gradually stronger, and soon that one eye will be better to you than my two to me." Just so it happened; and the baron, restored to sight and health, hunts, rides, and shoots with the best.

GOUT.—The sister of a friend of Professor Mundé's had been afflicted for a long time with pains in the foot and leg. She had sought relief in many remedies, and had tried the baths at Toplitz, without effect, and the disease was rather increased by them to such an extent that she could not walk. She had heard of the cold water cure; and once, when a paroxysm came on, she thought a foot-bath might relieve her, and determined to try it. From the very first she took she was able to walk, and in a few days was quite relieved of her complaint.—A clergyman came to Gräefenberg, whose gout in the feet and hands were so bad as to prevent his using them. After fifteen days' treatment at Gräefenberg, boils began to show themselves, a sure sign that the disease was being cured. He was obliged to return home by imperative business, even at the time of the crisis; but having the good sense to continue the treatment at his own house, he was not only completely cured of the gout, but also of an asthma which he had for a long time been labouring under.—A gentleman, high in station, had been for six years a martyr to the gout, which, after flying about his body, finished by settling in the feet, which were dreadfully inflamed and red to an excess. The doctors ordered him foot-baths in warm water, with a hot fomentation of plants, which increased the pain to such an alarming extent, that in despair the patient sought for relief in cold water, and found it instantly in a certain degree. On this, he repeated the cold water foot-baths, and began to think there might be something in the cold water treatment. Little more need be said : he was soon at Gräefenberg, where, from his age, 65, he was treated rather carefully, being placed in the wet sheet only, and not taking the douche. In other respects he was treated in the usual manner, and at the end of two months a radical cure was effected.

RHEUMATISM.—The parents of a little girl, aged seven years, finding that from the time she was one year old she had suffered from pains in the chest, which no medical treatment could alleviate, determined at last to bring her to Gräefenberg. M. Priessnitz at once declared the complaint to be rheumatism, and undertook to cure it. He wrapped the child in a wet sheet (renewed often during the day), and washed her each time it was changed in tepid water. This treatment soon brought on the usual fever, which is in itself a portion of the curative process. The parents began to be alarmed at its continuance; and remembering that they had been told by their physician to take her away from Gräefenberg if the treatment there increased the disease, resolved to take her home on the instant. To do this, however, they had to send for a carriage, which occupied the day. In this time the crisis ended; and when the parents came back they found their child playing in the fields! Of course they persevered in the treatment, and the little patient's health was soon perfectly restored.—A clergyman returning from a christening, where he had indulged in a good dinner, caught cold on an overcharged stomach. This brought on rheumatic pains in his arms and back, which no doctors could cure, and he was obliged to bear them without alleviation for one whole year. At last, patience being worn out, to Gräefenberg he came, where drinking cold water, perspiring and bathing, for three weeks, threw out an eruption all over his body, and eased him of his pain. The eruption and an asthmatic affection of the breathing were soon cured by a continuance of the treatment.—A cavalry officer of distinguished rank and services, was obliged to leave the army from asthmatic pains. He tried the water cure at home, and soon was induced by it to come to Gräefenberg. He stopped fifteen months, was thoroughly cured, and was able again to join his regiment.

SCIATICA.—A doctor, whose left leg had been for five years afflicted, came to Gräefenberg. After three months, boils broke out all over his legs, and laid him up in the house. After some time the boils discharged and healed, and then the doctor walked away quite cured.

DEAFNESS.—A gentleman caught cold on leaving the theatre, and lost the senses of hearing, smelling, and tasting. An abscess broke out near the ear after three months' treatment, and he was quite cured.

Professor Mundé describes the following cases of cure as coming under his own personal observation:—

CURE OF GOUT.—"The sister of a friend of mine, residing near Toplitz, suffered a long time pains in the foot and leg; she tried many remedies, besides the baths of Toplitz, without the slightest benefit; it even increased the disease to that degree that she could not walk. A violent paroxysm came on, during which she imagined the use of cold water might do her good: the first foot-bath that she took enabled her to walk; encouraged by this success, she renewed it, and was in a few days completely rid of the complaint. I saw her two years after, and heard her say she had not the slightest remains of her disease."

FEVER CURE.—"Soon after my arrival there, I was attacked by a strong fever. I first took a foot-bath, then a sitz-bath, wherein I remained for an hour. A friend of mine, seeing the fever augment, and my face get quite red, was frightened, and ran to Priessnitz, who came to see me at nine o'clock at night; he immediately placed me in a wet sheet, which was renewed in half an hour. I remained in it for an hour, during which time I slept, as Priessnitz had predicted; after which I was washed with cold water, and again placed in the wet linen, where I soon began to perspire abundantly, and to feel much relieved; I then slept until three o'clock in the morning, when I was again washed, and replaced in the wet sheet. I then began to perspire once more, until six o'clock, when, covered with perspiration, I was plunged into a cold water bath, where I remained but a few moments. I then went out to take a walk, and returned at eight o'clock to the breakfast table, exempt of all fever, heat, or even weakness.—There is a case which did not occur to myself, but of which I was an eye-witness. A merchant was attacked by nervous fever and delirium. The illness began by a sensation of burning in the stomach, which soon caused sickness. He took a sitz-bath, which did him no good. As the headach and sickness augmented, he drank water until he vomited, which relieved him: nevertheless, in an hour (ten o'clock at night), the invalid became worse and lost his senses. In this state he ran all over the house, with a light in his hand. From time to time his reason returned, and he was astonished to find himself thus; but the delirium soon came on again: thus he passed the whole night. It was only at nine o'clock the next morning that Priessnitz, hearing of the event, came to see him; he found him in bed, his eyes staring, his mouth open, his tongue dry and burning, and totally deprived of his senses. Priessnitz immediately ordered a sitz-bath, in which the patient remained for half an hour, and had him rubbed with cold water. After this, the invalid was placed in a wet sheet, which was renewed every ten minutes; in an hour he took another sitz-bath for half an hour, and was again placed in a wet sheet. He soon began to perspire, and gave evident signs of being relieved. These operations were continued until evening, when his reason returned. He slept all night: in the morning he was in a great state of perspiration, but quite free from pain. At eight o'clock in the morning, he asked for something to eat, and received bread and milk; and for dinner he had a soup, made from meat, with barley in it. The remainder of the day was passed quietly; the second and third nights were passed nearly in the same way as the first. On the fourth day he tried to take a cold-bath, but was seized with shooting pains in the head; he therefore took a tepid bath at the temperature of 61° Fahrenheit. This illness began on the 8th of September. On the 14th of the same month, the invalid was out to dinner, at which he partook of everything he found upon the table. A few days after this he quitted Gräefenberg, perfectly cured. There had been a similar case at Gräefenberg a few days before my arrival, the termination of which was equally fortunate. I was informed of this by some invalids who had preceded me. Priessnitz says, that this disease, taken in the commencement, is easily and quickly cured; later, it requires more time. Nevertheless, whatever may have been its duration, cold water is always efficacious.

CANCER.—"One remarkable case which I witnessed at Grüefenberg was that of an invalid who had formerly suffered from a chancre in the mouth, which was cured, but the disease not eradicated. Some years after, an abscess formed on the left instep. After nine months of medical treatment, the doctors found that they could not prevent the disease entering the bone. It at length became so serious, that no other resource was left but amputation. This the invalid refused to submit to, saying he would go to Grüefenberg. The doctors endeavoured to dissuade him, but he persisted in his resolution, which, however, he only carried into execution after remaining nine months in the hospital, where he became a skeleton, and so weak that he could not walk a step. Three weeks after his arrival at Grüefenberg, he could walk with the assistance of a stick; the ulcer alluded to cured!! Another appeared on the right foot, which kept the invalid confined to his room six weeks. At length the cure was effected, and the ulcers disappeared altogether. One would scarcely believe that a patient, who was reduced to skin and bone, should, during this treatment, become so stout that his clothes would not fit him, notwithstanding his having perspired for some hours every day: yet such was the fact. There is nothing to fear in the cold water treatment; for although a quantity of the juices are lost by perspiration, they are more than replaced. By means of the enormous appetite possessed by all the invalids at Grüefenberg, they not only gain that which they have lost, but acquire new strength. This is not the case with any other method of perspiration. On the arrival of the invalid last alluded to, Priessnitz praised him for having refused to submit to amputation, which could not have cured him, the cause of his disease being syphilis. This case required altogether nine months to cure. This is certainly a long time; but previous to that, the invalid had passed the same time in an hospital, where, after being tortured by drugs, hot rooms, &c., his misery was rendered complete by the doctors declaring, that nothing remained but amputation.—A lady had a cancer in the breast: the disease continued to increase, in spite of all the remedies, internal and external applied; at last amputation was proposed, to which the invalid agreed. On seeing, the instruments, she fainted; the operation was postponed till the following day; in the interim, some one spoke of Grüefenberg, where she determined to go. After following the treatment at Grüefenberg for six weeks, the breast became so much better, that she returned home, where Priessnitz advised her to continue the cure, which was soon crowned with complete success."

CHOLERA.—"The inspector of a large village belonging to the Crown arrived at Graefenberg; he had been ill for six weeks, but being of a robust constitution, he had during that time resisted all symptoms of cholera excepting sickness. He was much astonished at being ordered to drink milk, and eat bread and butter, which he did at Priessnitz's, as he placed entire reliance on him. After this repast he returned to his room, where he found a sitz-bath at the temperature of about 55° Fahr., already awaiting him. He was still more astonished, when, after some minutes, a discharge of wind greatly relieved the pains of the stomach. On leaving the bath he went to bed, prior to which a heating bandage was placed on the stomach, and he slept until the following day. This was the first time of sleeping since the commencement of the disease. He was completely cured, and returned home quite well. To dissipate all doubts which might be raised on the nature of this disease, I shall add the recital of the invalid on his arrival at Grüefenberg. 'The cholera,' said he, 'ravaged the village which I inhabited. The inhabitants were terrified, and refused to assist the sick; they had also suspended all labour, expecting to die. Thinking it was my duty to set them an example, I visited all the sick, and touched those who were timid, to give them courage. This conduct produced the effect I had expected, but it gave me the cholera, for which I was immediately treated by a doctor of the village, but without finding any relief; from thence to Vienna, without any better success. Grüefenberg was my last resource; I went, and there regained my health."

"It is not advisable to bathe the whole body with cold water: strong constitutions could bear it, but it is to be feared that re-action would not follow in weak persons; if so, death would be inevitable. Fever is, as I have already said, the only danger to be feared in these diseases. It is its violence which closes the pores and prevents the breaking out of the eruptive matter. The way to moderate it, and facilitate the eruption, is as already described, the efficacy of which is daily sanctioned by experience. I will now mention three cures which, without medicine, and with nothing but cold water, I performed in my own family. The first is a case of measles in an adult; the two others are of scarlatina in my two young children."

MEASLES.—"My servant, 20 years of age, caught the measles. As she refused all remedies, I proposed to her, in order to quiet the fever, which was very strong, that she should be wrapped up in a wet sheet; having agreed to this, she soon began to perspire profusely; this determined me to leave her there for seven or eight hours; she was then washed with water at the temperature of 61° Fahrenheit. This first perspiration was followed by an abundant eruption of red spots, which covered the whole body. I repeated the same process the next day, when the fever completely ceased. The parents having learned how I was healing their daughter, immediately came to take her home, fearing that such a treatment might be attended with dangerous consequences. In twelve days the invalid came back to her service, assuring me that, whilst at home, she had taken no other remedy than cold water."

SCARLATINA.—"Two of my children, one eight years old, the other five, were attacked with scarlatina, the eldest first. He was wrapped up in a sheet, whilst my other children, as yet unattacked, were repeatedly immersed in cold water. In three days, the one five years of age became ill; no doubt because he had previously taken the infection. The others did not take it at all. The second little invalid kept his gaiety and appetite, and was not wrapped up in a wet sheet, but only washed all over, morning and evening. The fever with both was very moderate. All was going on according to my wishes, when my wife became so alarmed as to suspend the treatment for four days. The consequence was, that the fever soon redoubled its intensity, and the children were in such pain that they could not move. It was so violent at the back of the eldest's head, that inflammation of the brain was to be feared. By my wife's desire, who now saw the folly of her fears, I again began my treatment. This time I gave the invalid a sitz-bath, after which he was enveloped in a wet sheet, which I renewed every half-hour. He soon went to sleep: this sleep lasted two hours, and gave proof of the efficacy of my proceedings, and courage to myself to go on with sitz-baths and general fomentations. The regular order of the system being re-established, I replaced the invalid in his dry bed, where he slept for several hours. In two days all danger disappeared. On the tenth day of the disease, a total scaling of the skin came on. The invalid, excepting a little weakness, was perfectly cured. The illness of the youngest was so simple, that he only required ablutions. He kept his brother company during the whole of his illness. Three weeks after the commencement of this eruption, I took them out walking in cold weather, without the walk being followed by any bad consequences. I however must add, that two days previous to exposing the new, fine, and delicate skin to the fresh air, they were bathed, morning and evening, in cold water."

INFLAMMATION OF THE BRAIN.—" I shall now relate a miraculous cure which was performed by this process in the little town of Freiwaldau. A labourer fell from a height, and having fractured his skull, inflammation of the brain ensued, and the invalid was entirely given up by the doctor of the place. Priessnitz visited him, and the next day he came to his senses, and, after some time, was perfectly cured."

OPHTHALMIA, OR INFLAMMATION OF THE EYES.—" A captain thus attacked, felt, after several head-baths which he continued for three-quarters of an hour, a pungent pain in the head, accompanied by swelling of the ears. An abscess was expected in one of these organs, when the pain gave way to a virulent deposit, formed in the thick part of the cheek; after this, the eyes were re-established.—Another sufferer came to Graefenberg, with an exfoliation in the corner of the eye. To the whole of the treatment Priessnitz added eye-baths; after each of which the invalid was to look fixedly at the light, and immediately re-plunge the eyes into cold water. This man, who was perfectly blind on coming, was, on leaving Graefenberg, able to read with spectacles.—A third patient presented a very remarkable case of blindness, the result of a cold, caught during hunting, by which he lost his sight. He had been nine months blind, when he arrived at Graefenberg; after each process of perspiration which he submitted to twice a day, the bath and the head-bath, matter mixed with blood came from the eyes. One might say that some pounds exuded from the eyes in the course of three weeks. I did not see the termination of this cure, before leaving Graefenberg; but I can affirm, that the last time I spoke to the invalid, he could distinguish colours, and also objects at certain distances."

The following cases of cures Mr. Claridge in his work on hydropathy, states to have come under his own experience while at Graefenberg:—

SPINAL COMPLAINT.—" A Polish general, who had a complaint of the spine, on his arrival at Freiwaldau, was told by his friends who met him, as he descended from his carriage, that there was no doubt he would immediately throw away his crutches, and be perfectly cured if he followed the system. He sat talking with them on one of the seats outside the house; when M. Priessnitz came up on horseback, he rose to salute him; the latter begged him to be seated, and instantly said, 'I perceive that the water cure will not be available in your complaint.' The general afterwards said that M. Priessnitz recounted to him all his sufferings with the greatest exactness. The general, however, then answered, 'Well, I may as well die here, for I have tried all other remedies in vain; but the most painful part of the matter is, that I have a young family, which I had hoped to have lived to see brought up.' The other replied, 'Although cold water will not cure you, it will relieve your pains, enable you to dispense with crutches, and will prolong your life; but as you regard these as advantages, avoid drugs.' The general at once determined on residing there for some years. He is now cheerful, out of pain, and walks with the use of a stick. He is a personage of such importance that all visitors to Graefenberg will at once know to whom this anecdote alludes."

GOUT.—" A gentleman from Galicia, forty-five years of age, told me that he came here to consult Priessnitz, and take a few baths, in consequence of some indications of gout, which he suspected was coming on, on account of his having indulged that year in the gaieties of the carnival. The gentleman was here six years ago, stayed four months, and was perfectly cured of gout, with which he had been annoyed for many years, spring and autumn. M. Priessnitz assured him, that if he resorted to his former temperance, and used cold water, he would have no return of disease."

SORE LEGS.—" I knew three persons at Graefenberg whose disease had settled in their legs; in each case, amputation had been recommended by the faculty. These invalids have been at Graefenberg from fifteen months to two years, and all were nearly recovered when I left."

FEVER.—" One object that interested me very much, was a gentleman, supported by two crutches, and led by a servant. On inquiry, I found he was a medical man, from Sweden; that two days previous to the one when I saw him, he had had a fever; that during the day, M. Priessnitz had applied no less than eighteen wet sheets, and then the bath. In a week I was astonished to see this person going up to Gräfenberg with the use of only a stick; and in ten days more he was as upright, and walked as well, as anybody else."

GENERAL WEAKNESS.—" At a ball which takes place every week at Gräfenberg, I saw an aged female using two crutches, and supported by a servant. I was informed that this lady, previously to coming to Gräfenberg, had been confined four years, the first two years to her bed, and the last two years, not being able to support an horizontal position, had been supported day and night by pillows. She had only been here three weeks, and was then able to be brought into the ball-room. She made daily progress, and, when I left, was walking out of doors with the use of a stick. A lady, from general debility, was brought to Gräfenberg in a carriage, built on purpose, so that the sofa might be taken in and out. She told me for ten years she had not had the use of her legs: in two months, at Gräfenberg, she was walking about; though to eradicate the cause of her complaint, M. Priessnitz said she must stay twelve months. Not being a medical man, I do not know what disease this lady was labouring under."

"Any medical man," concludes Mr. Claridge, "who could have inquired into the different complaints of parties, might multiply cases almost *ad infinitum*; I merely give the above as coming within my own immediate observation, without having taken any means of collecting them."

We may conclude this part of our subject, by drawing attention to a report made to the Government by a distinguished medical man who presides at the head of one of the hydropathic establishments, maintained in Berlin at the expense of the state, which states that out of 280 patients who had been subjected to the cold water cure in 1840, there had been but one death (that of a child three years of age, who at the commencement was declared too far gone to give great hopes of its recovery.)

A FEW WORDS OF ADVICE IN CONCLUSION.

Convinced, as all must now be, of the salutary influence of cold water, it becomes only necessary, in conclusion, to give some details of the general rules of life and habits which all should observe, in order to assist and second, as far as in their power, the action of cold water upon the system. We shall, therefore, in this final portion of our work, endeavour to set forth, in a few words, what both experience and reason teach us to do daily for the preservation of our health.

On rising in the morning, the first thing to be done is to wash, all over, the head especially, with cold water; the mouth must be rinced first, and the teeth cleaned with cold water, then two or three glasses of spring water drunk; and, after this, the whole person washed. If a thickness in the throat be felt, gargle well, and rub the outside of the throat three or four times a-day, with the hand wetted in cold water; keep the water in the mouth as long as possible, and repeat it when it becomes warm. This plan is recommended for dispersing any obstruction of the throat, and strengthening its membranes. If you feel cold, this sensation will soon go off, after walking up and down the room a few times. After taking coffee or tea at breakfast, a glass of water will be found of great advantage in diminishing any of their exciting effects. A glass of water about an hour before dinner will sharpen the appetite and invigorate the digestion. As regards dinner, let excess be avoided, and the quality of the food requires then but little attention: let vegetables, however, be taken with the meat, which, alone, is of too nourishing a nature, and has a tendency to thicken the humours. Salt meat and spices are not to be taken, as they cause acidity, and bring on inflammatory diseases. Things taken too hot are injurious to the teeth and stomach. Animals refuse all hot drinks and food, and their example should be followed. Priessnitz recommends his patients neither to eat or drink anything hot; and, in complaints of the chest, allows nothing but cold food. At dinner, cold water is highly recommended as a beverage. If not thirsty it may be drank, even after dinner, in a sufficient quantity to dilute the chyle. There is no settled measure of quantity, as all depends upon each person's constitution, and each must do as best suits his own system. For ourselves, we take our water at dinner, increasing the quantity if the repast be any richer or more substantial than usual. We take from three to five glasses at dinner, and find it attended with the best results: we, therefore, should advise it as a rule for general adoption. Eat slowly, and chew well; food, as the proverb says, " if well masticated, is half digested." If, after dinner, you find too much has been eaten, take two or three glasses of spring water to aid digestion. Strong exercise, whether of mind or body, is to be avoided soon after dinner; custom, alone, in laborious occupations, renders this endurable without injury; but persons of delicate constitution or advanced age should repose themselves for an hour. Those, on the contrary, of sedentary habits, should walk about, either in the room or in the open air.

A glass of water before going to bed, and friction of the body with a damp cloth, will ensure a healthy sleep; and those who wish to preserve their health will go to bed at ten o'clock; for two hours' sleep before midnight are better than all the other hours: it is this early sleep by which people are able to get up early in the morning. The advantage of early rising need not be told here. A man in health will find five hours of unbroken sleep sufficient.

In winter, the rooms are not to be kept too warm, lest the contrast be too great in going out; and this observation applies also to dress, which though of course fitted to the season, should always be as light as possible. Those who use cold water daily will want no flannel-waistcoast, lamb's-wool stockings, or such encumbrances, which only weaken the skin, and make it too susceptible. The head itself, though before so sensitive to rheumatism or cold, after being washed with cold water, grows hardy, fears no draught, and wants no nightcap even while sleeping. But all depends not on cold water alone, and the liberal use of it. Wholesome air and free exercise are the great desiderata for the preservation of health and long life. Those who are most in the open air, as sportsmen, gardeners, gamekeepers, &c., we know by experience, live to the greatest age, and enjoy the most vigorous health. Let us, then, as far as is in our power, follow their example, and feed our systems, as much as possible, with the wholesome food of pure air, which only can be attained by exercise. Let us throw open our doors and windows, summer and winter, to air the rooms, nor suffer a day to pass without taking good exercise in walking, if our circumstances will not allow of our riding. Such exercise, and cold bathing, or washing, with water-drinking, will most effectually operate in protecting us from those diseases to which all who neglect them are most surely liable, inasmuch as they will render the human frame less sensitive to those changes of weather and temperature in which so many diseases have their origin.

HOW TO GO TO GRAEFENBERG.

The following are the routes to Grüefenberg as given by Mr. Claridge;—

ROUTES TO GRAEFENBERG.

First route.

The point to which the traveller from England ought first to direct his attention, is Dresden; to reach this he may proceed as follows:—

London to Ostend by steam-boat, fourteen hours; Ostend to Liege by rail-road, seven hours; Liege to Aix-la-Chapelle by diligence, one day (posting requires the same time); Aix-la-Chapelle to Cologne by railway, four hours; Cologne to Frankfort by steam-boat, *via* the Rhine, two days; Frankfort to Leipsic by diligence, thirty-six hours; Leipsic to Dresden by railway, seven hours. Thence, Dresden to Breslau by diligence, thirty-one hours; from Breslau to Niesse by diligence, nine hours; at Niesse a small carriage, with either one or two horses, may be engaged for Grüefenberg; to reach which about four hours will be required.

Second route.

London to Hamburgh, fifty to sixty hours; Hamburgh to Magdeburg, by steam-boat, two days; Magdeburg to Dresden, *via* Leipsic, by railway, eight hours. Or from Hamburgh, the traveller may take the diligence to Berlin, which makes the journey in thirty-six hours; and from thence to Dresden by railway, in twelve hours.

The outlay in actual travelling expenses, by either of these routes, without including provisions, will not exceed £10.

Third route.

Persons proceeding to Grüefenberg from the East *via* the Danube, or from Italy, should make a point of reaching Vienna, and from thence continue their journey by railway to Olmütz, which occupies half a day; sleep there, and hire a carriage for Grüefenberg: this forms the second day's journey. If they have occasion to stay, *en route*, they will find tolerable accommodation at Hansdorf, three hours'-distance from their place of destination.

It is expected that the railroad, the whole distance from Ostend to the Rhine, will be completed this year; and it is in contemplation to make a railroad from Frankfort to Leipsic, and another from Dresden to Breslau; so that the journey to Grüefenberg will be accomplished with very little fatigue, and in a short period of time.

The expenses of living at Grüefenberg are as follow:—

	£	s.	d.
Board, including breakfast, dinner, and supper (a week), 4 florins or	0	8	0
An apartment, 2 florins or	0	4	0
Baddiener, or bath-servant, 2 florins	0	4	0
	0	16	0
The lowest fees usually paid to M. Priessnitz is 2 florins, or 4s. a week	0	4	0
	£1	0	0

But here it must be observed that 2 florins or 4s. is the minimum ever offered to M. Priessnitz for his attendance; many increase it to double that sum, and others make handsome presents. However, it will be seen that a residence and medical attendance at Grüefenberg is necesarily only attended with an expense of £1 sterling per week. At Freiwaldau in the neighbourhood, a good lodging for a single person, of two rooms, in the best situation, may be had at from 5s. to 10s. a week. The usual price for dinner is 1s. For a family an apartment, consisting of three or four rooms, and a kitchen, will cost from 12s. to 20s. per week; after this a number of little articles must be purchased or hired; as the apartments are only furnished like those at Grüefenberg, all articles of consumption are remarkably cheap; for instance, beef and mutton are 3d. per lb., veal, 2½d., pork 3½d.; price of bread in proportion.